-16

menopause
breakthroughs

Grace Johnston

ROWAN COLLEGE
at Gloucester County
Library
1400 Tanyard Road
Sewell, NJ 08080

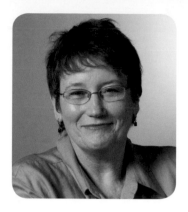

Based in Melbourne, Australia, author Grace Johnston says she enjoyed writing this book- and one of the main reasons was because she's reached an age where menopause has become academic. As a grandmother of four, Grace says she's more than happy to have it that way.

Grace was originally a journalist, and spent much of her later life working with people going through change; in organisations, as a counsellor and consultant working with mature aged jobseekers and as a pastoral carer in a major cancer hospital..

She is the author of a dozen books since her first was published in 2000 (*Aligning Your Work and Purpose*). These include the *What's Good for You* series, *You've Got the Job*, and *101 Ways to Get a Job*.

With thanks for the expertise and support of Jean Hailes for Women's Health.

Published by
Wilkinson Publishing Pty Ltd
ACN 006 042 173
Level 4, 2 Collins Street, Melbourne, Vic 3000
Tel: 03 9654 5446 www.wilkinsonpublishing.com.au

International distribution by Pineapple Media Limited
(wwwpineapple-media.com) ISSN 2200-013005

National Library of Australia Cataloguing-in-Publication entry:

Author:	Johnston, Grace, author.
Title:	Menopause breakthroughs / Grace Johnston.
ISBN:	9781922178701 (paperback)
Series:	WP health series.
Subjects:	Menopause. Menopause--Treatment. Women--Health and hygiene.
Dewey Number:	618.175

Photos and illustrations by agreement with international agencies, photographers and illustrators from iStockphoto.

Design: Jo Hunt
Printed in China

Contents

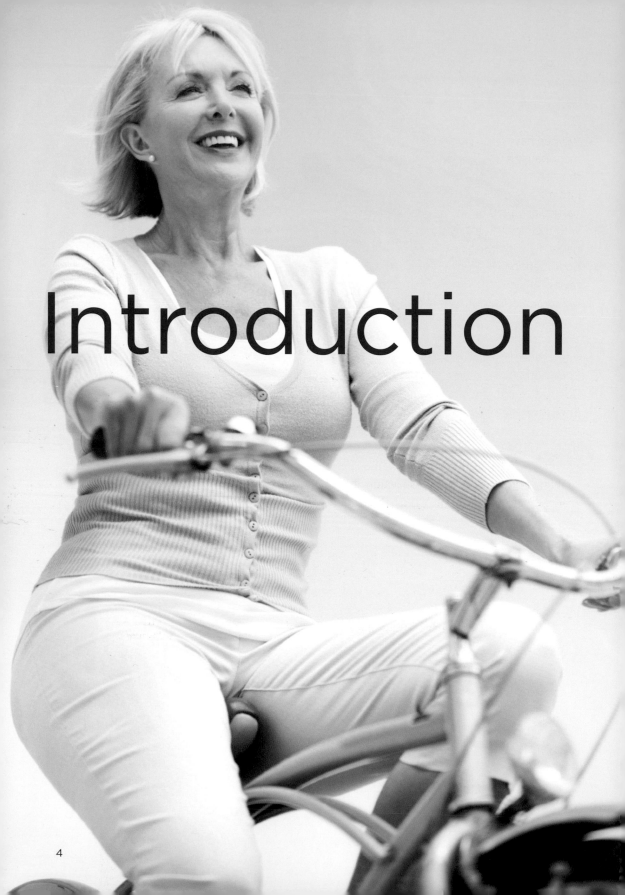

Introduction

Welcome to this second edition of *Menopause Essentials*, now called *Menopause Breakthroughs*.

Women have been going through menopause since time immemorial, but in the last few years research has continued into methods to help those women particularly hard hit by this life change cope with their symptoms; and assist women generally with living healthy lives during and post-menopause. Hence, we thought we'd review the latest findings and include these in this new edition.

You'll also find an updated section on menopause and super foods, and, up the back, some great recipes for eating well during and after menopause.
The word *menopause* comes from two Greek root words, *men*, which means month, and *pausis*, cessation, and, of course, refers to the ending of a woman's monthly period cycle, or menstruation. It marks the end of a woman's reproductive life. During menopause a woman's ovaries stop producing hormones, and in particular oestrogen, and the release of eggs capable of being fertilised ceases.

While the word menopause in fact refers to the last ever period, we use it colloquially in a more general sense to cover the complex process leading up to, and sometimes beyond the last period.

This can be a challenging time not just for women, but for their partners and families – and even at times workmates. For women it's the end of their potential to be mothers and, while for some that's a relief, for others it can be a time of considerable sadness. Our self-image changes and the view in the mirror may come to differ markedly from how we feel inside.

But menopause is a natural part of ageing and one of life's major times of transition for women. Many simply pass through it with few symptoms. For a lucky few, periods simply stop and the symptoms their less fortunate sisters complain of pass them by all together.

Fact

20 per cent of women experience no symptoms at all during menopause and another 60 per cent have only mild symptoms.

In days gone by, women simply put up with the symptoms. I remember coming home from school one day and finding my mother collapsed on the floor; it was years later I was told this had been blamed on her 'time of life', and that she would just have had to put up with such things until she had passed through 'the change' and reached the other side.

Well, we have options today; lots of options. So many options, in fact, that confusion and anxiety can replace resignation ... Should I try hormone replacement therapy? How does it work and is it safe? What about all that bad press it received a few years ago; is it a breast cancer risk? Do natural alternatives work? Are they safe and, if I choose to use them, should I tell my doctor about them? What about bioidentical hormones; what are they, how do they work and are they safe? And so on.

In *Menopause Breakthroughs* we endeavour to explore and answer some of these questions. In this process we'll draw on a wide range of research and expertise from around the world, but in particular I want to acknowledge and say *thanks* to the wonderful staff and highly qualified and experienced expert consultants at Jean Hailes for Women's Health, the headquarters of which is based in Melbourne, Australia.

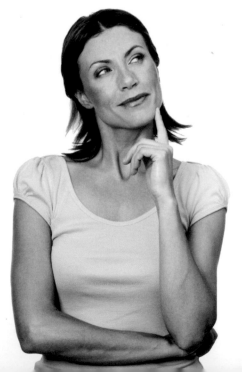

Three things to note:

- I'm using British English spelling and Australian terminology, and occasionally this may be at odds with what you may be familiar with. I trust that doesn't offend!

- In Western countries we tend to use the one word, 'menopause', to cover the time up to and including a woman's last ever period. The medical fraternity, however, uses the word perimenopause or menopause transition for the years or months leading up to 'menopause', which they use to mean the last period that ends menstruation. Perimenopause, then, is the time when many women start to experience various effects of the hormone changes going on in the body – hot flushes, night sweats etc, though these also can affect life after menopause as well. We will sometimes use the word 'perimenopause', but will mostly use the one word 'menopause', to describe whole menopausal transition from having a regular menstruation cycle to the final episode of menstruation to a post-menopause, post-reproductive life. This is the way, after all, that most people think and talk; and

- While we've been careful to check all the information included in this book, please do your own research as well, and seek expert advice from appropriately qualified practitioners.

Before we start, I'd like to pass on some information given to me when I was around 42-43 years old by a wonderful woman in her late fifties. At the time I did not know what she was talking about, but her words have stayed with me over the years since.

She was a naturopath and was one of the most vibrant and beautiful women I have ever come across. She said to me:

"Grace, don't ever be afraid of the menopause. Women think it's the end of their lives, but believe me, it's just the beginning of a whole new and wonderful stage. You'll find you'll be so much freer to be yourself and you will no longer care what people think about you. And best of all, is that all that energy you used to need keeping your monthly cycles going now becomes available for other things – and you can choose how you use it. Believe me, the years post-menopause are the most wonderful time of life of all!"

Well, now I'm definitely in my post-menopause years and I can honestly say this naturopath was right; these for me are proving to be, in many ways, the best, happiest and most productive time of my life.

I'll just finish with sharing an image with you, the reader. I find I am able now to put this menopausal stage of life in perspective, and when I do that sort of thing often an image pops into my mind. In this case, the image is of a veil being lifted off me, allowing me somehow to see everything in my life more clearly. The veil was held in place for many years by all those reproductive hormones, but now energy and life focus are back, in bucket loads.

My hope is that you too may find this is so when your turn comes.

Grace Johnston

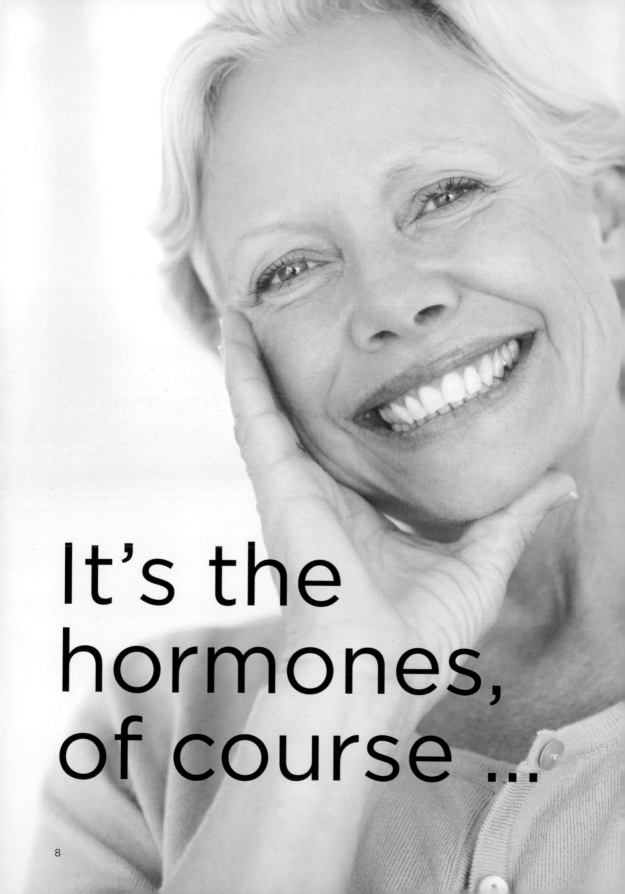

It's the hormones, of course ...

What's new?

Nothing much is new, although there's lots of research being conducted in labs around the world.

Q 1: Is menopause all about our hormones?

The answer is probably, 'yes, mostly...'

Women's hormones have a bad reputation. It's our hormones, after all, which seem to take the blame every time we have an off day, a bad mood, become irritated by someone or perhaps do something that seems out of character. And that's even before we get to those years of the menopause when our hormones and our lives go through major change!

Like most stereotypes, this characterisation of our hormones carries some truth, but women are not alone when it comes to having hormones govern our everyday life. It may come as a surprise to many men, but they have hormones too and these have a profound effect on their lives. We look at men and menopause in some detail later.

Menopause is a time in a woman's life when there's a major change in how hormones function within our bodies. It's a natural event. It's happened for women who lived long enough since time immemorial. At some time in every woman's life, usually between 45 and 55, she will experience her last period. That, by definition, is menopause. The average age of menopause for women in Western countries is 51.

Q 2: How is menopause diagnosed?

Before a formal diagnosis of menopause can be made, a women needs to have lived for one year free of periods. There are some exceptions, which we'll come to shortly.

Because periods can become quite irregular in the months, and sometimes even years, leading up to the very last period, it can be hard to pinpoint when we've just had the very last one. So it's hard for us to know when to throw a party, or go into mourning, as the case may be!

This lead-up time goes by the name of 'menopause transition', or 'perimenopause'. While these are the medical terms for the stage leading up to periods ceasing, in ordinary everyday language we tend to call the whole process 'menopause'.

Q 3: What starts the whole process going in the first place?

A woman's perimenopause is prompted when the levels of two key hormones start fluctuating. These hormones are oestrogen and progesterone and their levels can swing rapidly from very high to very low without apparent reason.

Oestrogen and progesterone, the main female sex hormones, are present in baby girls at birth but they are kept 'switched off' until a girl reaches puberty. This is when the hypothalamus gland starts releasing increasing amounts of gonadotropin-releasing hormone, or GnRH. The hypothalamus, situated deep within the brain and a little above the pituitary gland, is often referred to as the body's 'master gland'. It plays a controlling role in many of the body's functions, in men as well as women.

The release of GnRH prompts a woman's pituitary gland to then release a couple of other hormones - luteinising hormone (LH) and follicle-stimulating hormone (FSH). These in turn then cause the ovaries to start their hormone production.

While GnRH, LH and FSH are not household names, the main hormones produced by the ovaries in response to them – oestrogen and progesterone – are certainly better known. Most of us would think of oestrogen, for example, as the female hormone.

We women owe a great deal to oestrogen, good and bad. It's the hormone mainly responsible for our breasts developing and for our reproductive organs – vagina, uterus and Fallopian tubes – growing and maturing. We can blame it too for some of the fat that settles around our hips, thighs and bottoms! It has a lot to do with our feelings of wellbeing, too.

When a girl's born, her two ovaries contain an estimated 1,000,000 ovarian follicles each. Each follicle contains a circle of cells surrounding an immature egg – and therein lies the potential for new life. By the time a girl reaches puberty and her oestrogen levels ramp up, many of these follicles will have been absorbed into the body, leaving her with some 400,000 or so immature eggs. That's more than enough, you would think, to get pregnant many times over by the time menopause comes along!

Odd Spot

Though women are born with maybe a million eggs in each ovary, we only release some 400-500 mature ones in all the years between puberty and menopause. By the time we hit menopause, it's unlikely there are any left capable of reaching maturity and being fertilised.

Q 4: How is oestrogen produced?

Oestrogen is produced by the cells within the follicles that surround the immature eggs, and one of its roles is to cause a thickening of the lining of the womb each month, in anticipation of pregnancy.

When this fails to happen the body releases this lining – a process we refer to as having a period, or menstruation.

The second important hormone, progesterone, is released as part of the process of an egg coming to maturity and being released at ovulation.

Although only one of a woman's many, many eggs (in almost most cases, anyway) reaches sufficient maturity to be released at ovulation each month, quite a few others begin the process. So, while a woman has one egg ready for fertilisation, perhaps another 10-20 ovarian follicles have been used up. These are absorbed back into the body.

This means that, over time, the number of available immature eggs decreases significantly, leading to a decline in hormone production ... and so we come to perimenopause, or the lead-up to menopause.

Q 5: What changes to my periods will the start of menopause cause?

As oestrogen production declines, women are likely to experience such things as:

- Irregular periods. The time between them may be longer, or shorter, or sometimes longer and sometimes shorter, so knowing when to expect the next one turns into a bit of a mystery;
- Shorter periods. You may find a period lasts only a day or two;
- Lighter flow. Sometimes a period can hardly seem to have been worth the trouble!
- Longer periods and stop-start periods. Where once you might have got away with 4 or 5 days, now it might be twice that long ... and sometimes even longer. Or you might think you've finished, only to find the flow starting again a day or so later;
- Heavier flow. Enough said.

Note: *if you're experiencing heavy or prolonged bleeding, best to see your doctor or alternative therapist. A couple of reasons: firstly, it may be a sign of something else going on and secondly, excess blood loss can be debilitating.*

Q 6: Is there a normal age for menopause?

The answer to this question depends on where you live in the world.

A 2008 study found the average age in the developed world is 51.4 years. Other studies have put 50-51 years as the average age for women in the USA, Iran, Italy and Slovenia, while women in Taiwan, Korea, Singapore, Lebanon, Turkey, Greece, Mexico and Morocco are likely to reach menopause a little earlier – from age 47 to 50.

Q 7: So how would you define early menopause?

It's quite hard to define early menopause compared to menopause, as there's a great deal of natural variation amongst women. For example, many women in Western countries reach menopause between 40 and 45, which is considered early but not abnormal.

If a woman experiences menopause before 40, she is said to have had *premature* menopause. There may be several reasons for such an early cessation of periods, including:

- A natural decline in hormone production. Perhaps one in 100 women reaches menopause before 40 for no known reason. This goes by the name of 'premature ovarian failure', or 'premature ovarian insufficiency' and it isn't yet fully understood. It may have something to do with genetic factors or autoimmune diseases.
- Surgical removal of ovaries for medical reasons, or
- As a side effect of chemotherapy or radiotherapy for cancer treatment.

Q 8: How then would you define late menopause?

The occasional woman is still menstruating naturally at 58-59, and even at 60, but it is very rare. Most women have reached menopause by 55, which is still considered at the upper end of the 'normal' age range.

Q 9: How long can I expect it to last?

Again, some women seem to draw the short straw and others the long one.

For a lucky few it will be just a few months, but the average is four years. Some women find they suffer symptoms for a good 10 years, and the odd woman finds herself experiencing the occasional hot flush well into old age.

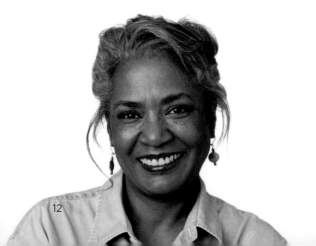

Q 10: You mentioned different countries before – were you implying that a woman's experience of menopause depends on what country she lives in?

As we have seen, the average age of menopause differs across countries, so it may well be possible to conclude, as some anthropologists have done, that cultural differences affect menopause.

Studies by anthropologist Marcha Flint[1] in the 1970s found very few women in a region of India complained of menopause symptoms at all. Her research was completed with 483 middle age Indian women of the Rajput caste in Rajasthan and Himachal Pradesh.

She ended up proposing the idea that these women didn't complain because they saw menopause as the key to a significant improvement in their social standing. Where previously during their fertile years these women were generally kept secluded from male company, after menopause they could freely mix in the company of men. So, menopause brought them greater freedom and recognition.

Flint also identified other cultures across the world – Africa, Micronesia, Nepal and the Tiwi Islands off the north of Australia – where women experienced a similar improvement in freedom and status.

She contrasted this with Western countries, with our emphasis on beauty and 'eternal youth'. This glorification of youth can lead women to fear menopause, suspecting they'll become 'invisible' and devalued. The subtle unconscious message of the West, fostered by the images of youth, health, slimness and beauty that bombard us every day, is that menopause marks a turning point that leads to the death of sexuality and ultimately to death.

Q 11: So you're saying menopause isn't the end?

To answer that I'm going to draw on the valuable resources – a list of Menopause Myths – produced by the Jean Hailes for Women's Health organisation.

MYTH – Menopause is the beginning of the end.
FACT – Menopause is a time of transition – while some women have negative feelings about the end of their reproductive years, others look forward to the next stage of their lives. Who you are, what your life experiences have been and how you feel about your life will all influence the way you experience menopause.

The attitude that you have toward this time of your life can influence your coping abilities, your emotional wellbeing and your risk of mood disorders. It is helpful to understand how you feel about the different areas of your life, along with the physical changes of menopause.[2]

Odd Spot

A 78-year-old Chinese woman is said to have conceived naturally in 2006 to become the oldest known mother in recorded history, while a 70-year-old Indian woman delivered twins in 2008 following invitro fertilisation treatment.

But for those of us who don't want to break records, the message is caution is better than confidence – at least for a while!

Q 12: Can I get pregnant after menopause?

Unfortunately it happens ever so occasionally in the menopausal years – so be cautious.

Defining the end of menstruation is tricky, given that periods become very irregular. So doctors advise continuing the use of contraception after what you assume to be your last period for at least two years if you're under 50, and for one year if you're over that age.

Menopause – not called 'change of life' for nothing

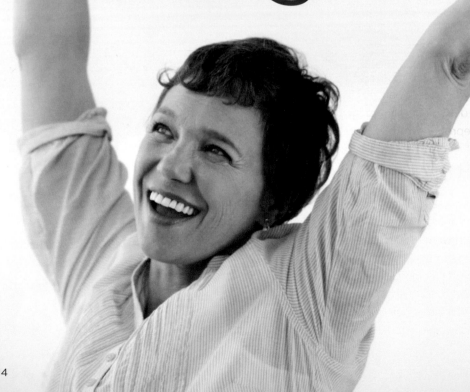

What's new?

- Again, nothing much; menopause has been part of a woman's life since time immemorial.
- Then again, it is much researched, so watch for regular media announcements.
- Research continues on a possible new test to predict menopause onset.

Q 13: I seem to remember menopause being referred to simply as 'the change' when I was young. Am I remembering correctly?

I think you're right; when I was growing up in country Australia in the 1950s, nobody used the word 'menopause'. Like most things to do with bodily functions, such as sex and reproduction, it was not polite in this country to talk about it, or at least not in front of the children.

Menopause was referred to euphemistically as 'change of life' or simply 'the change', and women were required simply to go through it. As there was little of the physiological knowledge or range of medical and other help available, that's what most women did – they 'went through it'.

And for some 80 per cent or so of women, that wasn't a problem – their menopausal symptoms, mild or severe, were just something they put up with and they got on with life. The other lucky few, as now, sailed through the whole change without any difficulties.

"I just woke up one morning, and I swear, without warning my breasts were a size bigger and I had fat around my stomach that hadn't been there the day before, and nothing helped me shift any of it. And then the hot flushes started, and the night sweats. My husband's asleep with an electric blanket on and I've kicked all but my sheet off!

"I think I felt angry with everyone and everything for a whole year, and when I wasn't angry I was crying for no reason at all. I'm not as angry now.

"But I'm not going to resort to taking anything. I've never believed in putting medicines into my body unless it's absolutely unavoidable, and I've made up my mind I just have to live through this. I just wish I knew how long it was going to take, though."
Jen, mid-50s, Melbourne

Q 14: What sort of symptoms can I expect in the lead up to menopause?

Menopausal symptoms, as set out above, affect some 80 per cent of women. For three in four these will be mild, relatively speaking of course. The other unlucky one in four will experience such severe symptoms that their lives are totally disrupted by them. An unfortunate few will experience the odd symptom, like hot flushes, at various times for the rest of their lives.

The best-known symptoms are:
....

- hot flushes, or hot flashes as they are called in the United States
- irregular periods and changes in menstruation
- night sweats
- vaginal dryness
- reduced libido (that is, interest in and desire for sex), as well as vaginal dryness leading to uncomfortable intercourse
- sore breasts
- aches and pains, particularly in the joints
- tiredness
- irritability and mood swings
- the 'blues' or even depression
- crawling or itching under the skin
- headaches
- urinary frequency
- sleeping difficulty
- memory lapses
- easy weight gain

Q 15: That's enough surely! Please don't tell me there's more?

Some less well-known symptoms include irregular heartbeat, dizziness, digestive problems and even a change in body odour!

Alongside all this, a woman may also find herself losing her self-esteem, particularly if previously she has placed great value on and drawn confidence from her role as a sexually attractive woman. That's not to say, of course, that a woman stops being sexually attractive at menopause, certainly not!

Q 16: People talk most about hot flushes, but what happens when we go through one?

The term *hot flushes* describes the sensation of warmth that spreads through the body and then dies away again. Women feel it particularly in the upper body – around the face and the neck. A vasomotor reaction is taking place, that is, the blood vessels close to the skin are responding to messages from the brain. In this case the blood vessels respond by dilating.

For some women it's like a subtle alteration of temperature that swiftly readjusts itself after a minute or two; for others it's like a raging fire that causes them to break out into a sweat.

Sweating and reddened skin let the world know we're going through menopause, even if we're keen to hide the fact. With menopause, there's no place to hide! Some unlucky women have reported having as many as 50 hot flushes in a day, but for most women they are just an occasional happening. It depends largely on how gradually or abruptly the body's hormone levels are changing.

Hot flushes are not known for their sense of timing ... They can arrive in the middle of an important business meeting, as you're in a tense interview with your child's teacher or while sitting by the pool drinking a martini. In each case, it's a matter of hanging in until they pass.

Q 17: Why is this happening?

A hot flush begins in the brain with the master gland, the hypothalamus. It regulates body temperature and, for some reason, the thermostat changes in midlife. It seems to be reset to a lower temperature than normal. Our bodies respond with a hot flush. This helps the body rid itself of this excess heat and energy. For some women this process is followed by feeling chilled as sweat evaporates and the body's temperature re-adjusts.

Make sure you dress in layered clothing so it's easy to take something off, or put something extra on as the temperature dictates. It helps to avoid hot and spicy food and alcohol and to drink more water. It's also worth working on stress and anxiety levels just to see if there's a link.

I've known women who get very business-like about their hot flushes and keep a diary for a week or two, noting when and where they occurred and any likely triggers. Whatever helps is what I say.

One woman tells it how it is

"I can't believe these hot flushes ... I feel like they suck the life out of me. My face gets red and the sweat pours down and I can feel my earlobes burning! I can feel my heart pounding and even the ends of my feet and fingers feel hot. Sometimes this lasts about a minute but the worst of them can go on for what seems like an eternity. Not much fun when I'm trying to act like a professional in a management team meeting at work! I can't wait until it's all over, even if I find I don't feel like a real woman any more."
Elinor – 50, North London, UK

The unfortunate truth is that as a rule hot flushes don't stop when a woman has had her last period. They are likely to continue for at least a year, more likely two, afterwards.

Q 18: I have a friend who claims she now wakes up each night in a hot sweat? What's going on for her?

Your friend is suffering from night sweats, which are the nocturnal variety of hot flushes. It's common for some women to find sleep disrupted by waves of heat followed by chills, together with feeling nauseated and having an irregular heart beat, though not all women who experience hot flushes are bothered by these last two night-time visitors.

Sweats can range in severity from so mild they don't even wake a woman up to so intense that they interrupt sleep and affect how a woman feels the next day. In fact night sweats go some (but not all) of the way to explaining other menopause symptoms such as tiredness, memory lapses and irritability.

The occasional woman experiences such severe night sweats that she wakes to find she's saturated with sweat to the point where she has to change her nightclothes and bed linen.

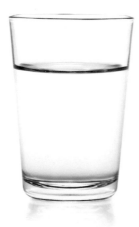

Another woman's story

"I am 46 years old, and I thought I was too young for any of this, but night sweats have been part of my life for the past 10 years. For the last 12 months, though, it's become really bad. I hardly ever get through a night without waking with my nightclothes wet, and most nights I also have to get up to go to the toilet. My periods have also become very irregular. I never know where I am; I may skip a month or have two or three periods in another month. My periods are lasting longer now, up to eight or nine days. Sometimes I'll stop for two or three days, then start again. It's making my life extremely stressful."
Susan, Cornwall, UK

Q 19: Can anything be done to help?

There are some common sense changes women can make that may help – sleeping in a cool environment and not too close to one's partner are obvious moves. So too are avoiding hot baths or saunas before bed, and changing a diet high in hot and spicy food and alcohol to one containing 'cooler' foods and drinking more water. It's also worth working on stress and anxiety levels just to see if there's a link.

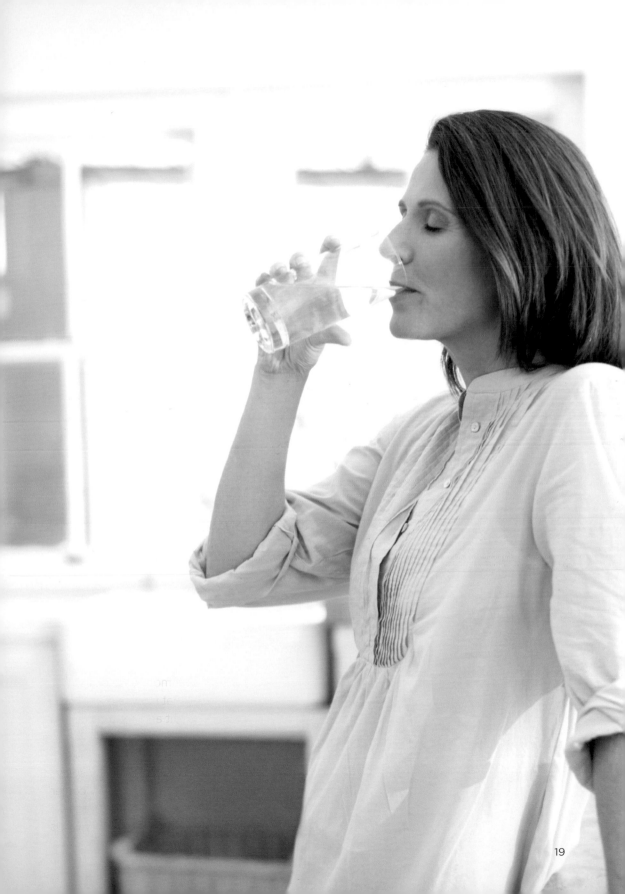

It's around now, when the night sweats kick in, that many women who planned to avoid medical interventions for menopause, start on hormone replacement.

Menopause is as individual as each woman who goes through it, so it's worthwhile for every woman to take note of her own experience and see if she can work out whether daytime factors are triggering this unpleasant night-time activity.

Odd Spot

Asian women report being less likely to experience night sweats than women from the West, and women of African origin are both more likely to have night sweats and to report them as severe than any other group.

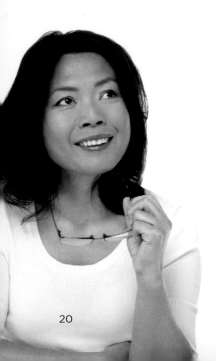

Q 20: Can you give advice on some of the other menopausal symptoms you listed previously – in particular menstruation changes and incontinence?

If you're not the 10 per cent of women who fly through perimenopause then this time of life may be full of surprises for you!

While a 28-day menstrual or period cycle is usual for most women, many naturally have regular cycles of shorter or longer duration. The hormone imbalances in the lead-up to menopause will almost inevitably cause this cycle to fluctuate, both in timing and flow. So, you may find yourself with another period only two to three weeks after the last one, or not for five weeks or more. One period may be very light; another may be so heavy it goes on for six or seven days or more and cause you significant inconvenience. Then, there may be clotting and unaccustomed cramping.

You may skip a period altogether and then come back to a normal cycle for a few months ... It can all be a bit of a roller coaster. The best advice is 'be prepared' – both for the start of an unexpected period and in terms of your use of contraception.

Recent research shows shortened intervals between periods are the most common change to the menstrual cycle during perimenopause.

Q 21: Okay, so what's the 'good news' on incontinence then?

I don't blame you for thinking incontinence is another topic we don't really want to talk about, let alone face.

Consultant gynaecologist Dr Elizabeth Farrell AM, former president of both the Australasian Menopause Society and the Asia Pacific Menopause Federation and Founding Director at Jean Hailes for Women's Health has some advice – and that is that we need to get over our embarrassment. She says effective incontinence treatment is available, and it's a misconception that bladder and bowel problems are just a part of normal ageing, and therefore simply to be put up with.

Our lessening ability to produce oestrogen is the culprit that has many post-menopausal women reluctant to laugh heartily, cough or sneeze. Many of us know from experience we may not be able to control the leaking of urine that follows. Lowered oestrogen levels cause a thinning of the tissues and ligaments that provide support for the bladder. Some 37 per cent of all women are affected by urinary incontinence to some degree.

Dr Farrell advises women to get their pelvic floor exercises going, and to adopt the view that exercising the pelvic floor muscles is as important as exercising other parts of their bodies.

"You may need to do pelvic floor exercises to improve the symptoms and, with a vaginal oestrogen cream absorbed into the local tissues, this may be enough to improve incontinence problems significantly", she says.

Dr Farrell also advises women not to cut down on drinking water in the hope this will reduce their incontinence. It has the opposite effect, she claims, because dehydration causes the bladder to become more irritated, causing a woman to want to 'go' more often, rather than less.

Odd Spot

It helps to keep your sense of humour ...

Several years ago my daughter took me to see a wonderful live show in Melbourne. Unfortunately I can't remember the full name (!), but it was all about menopause. A wonderful group of mature women sang and danced and made merry about menopause and all the treats that lie in store for women as we reach 'the change'.

The theatre was filled with older women (and the odd brave man) who understood all about menopause, incontinence, hot flushes, floppy bellies and comfy slippers etc, and it was totally liberating to recognise other women's experiences as well as my own and to laugh out loud. The other enjoyable aspect was to be with a group of women who shared the experience, understood the jokes, and were prepared to laugh at themselves and the whole menopausal thing.

Q 22: How can I know what's normal for me?

Let's call on the Jean Hailes expertise again:

MYTH – Bleeding for more than seven days is quite normal.

FACT – Forty per cent of women with heavy periods (menorrhagia is the medical term) think their bleeding is normal. Some five per cent of women aged between 30 and 49 see a gynaecologist because of menorrhagia.

ADVICE – It's abnormal for a woman to bleed more than one-third of a cup of blood over the course of a normal period, and bleeding for more than seven days is also abnormal. Either of these happenings – heavy bleeding and extended bleeding – can interfere with living a normal life during menopause because of the inconvenience, but also because they lead to iron deficiency, fatigue and lethargy.

Irregular or heavy periods are a definite sign that a woman is entering perimenopause. They can, however, also be a sign of various medical problems, including polyps, fibroids, hyperplasia or cancer. Hyperplasia is the name given to an increase in cells in normal tissue and can be a precursor of uterine cancer. So, don't put up with heavy bleeding for too long before you seek help.[3]

Q 23: Can I predict how long this menopause process is going to last?

Some medical experts offer women a blood test that measures levels of Follicle Stimulating Hormone and oestradiol, on the understanding that, by measuring these levels, it's possible to evaluate how long until they experience their final period. Oestradiol is the most important form of oestrogen found in a woman's body.

According to one internationally-renowned menopause expert, such tests are a 'waste of time'.

Professor Henry Burger is well equipped to comment. He's an endocrinologist and founding director of Jean Hales for Women's Health, and a former president of the International Menopause Society and Australasian Menopause Society. He's also an Honorary Professorial Fellow at the School of Medicine at Melbourne's Monash University (Australia).

Professor Burger says prediction tests are ineffective because hormone changes are unpredictable and vary from menstrual cycle to menstrual cycle. Research is currently being undertaken into the use of another hormone, anti-Müllerian hormone or AMH, as a potential predictor. Dr Burger says the hope is this may prove more accurate and reliable, but the research still needs more refining.

So, at this stage, perhaps your best predictor is still how long your mother's perimenopausal transition took, and the age at which it occurred.

When I was a young girl, many years ago, there was an old wives' tale which went something along these lines ... 'the earlier you start menstruation, the later you reach menopause'. I know I can vouch for this being the case for me, but that's hardly scientific verification. But, like many old wives' tales, this little saying may well contain a kernel of truth.

We listed several conditions before that affect the uterus and interrupt a woman's menstrual cycle. These included fibroids, cysts, polyps and endometriosis. Eating disorders and irritable bowel syndrome can also be added to the list, as can problems with the thyroid gland and suffering from anaemia.

Then there are some other obvious causes, such as a late pregnancy, having miscarried a baby, or recently having had a D & C, or to use its full name, a dilation and curettage.

Q 24: Is there a real danger of pregnancy at this time?

The answer is yes, but you'd have to be unlucky. It's quite common for women at this time of life to have periods, but not to ovulate in between. This is called anovulation – the ovaries do not release an egg, but periods still take place.

Because you can't tell for yourself whether an egg is released or not, best not to take any chances.

Q 25: Might there be other reasons my periods have become irregular?

Again, the answer is 'yes'. There are some health conditions, as well as some lifestyle factors, that can upset the menstrual cycle – at any age.

Q 26: Anything else I should know?

On the lifestyle front, over-exercise can cause periods to become very irregular, and putting on – or losing – lots of weight may also have an effect. Breast-feeding is another obvious menstrual cycle interrupter, but many a baby has been conceived when parents relied on that as a contraceptive! Stress, not eating properly, some medications and other illegal drugs, too much alcohol and caffeine – the list goes on.

But if you're in your forties or early fifties, the odds are that you've become irregular because you're perimenopausal.

Q 27: When should I see a medical practitioner?

This is up to you; you may want to make an appointment as soon as you notice your periods have changed and some of the other symptoms have kicked in. The diagnosis is usually fairly obvious, and is made from the history. Blood tests to check hormone levels are generally unreliable and are best avoided.

Your health professional is also a good source for general information on how best to manage your way through this major change in your life. Some symptoms warrant an immediate check-up, as we indicated before. Just as a reminder, these include blood clots, cramping and excessively heavy or very frequent periods.

Q 28: What happens to my body after menopause?

Unfortunately, stopping menstruation – the final period – doesn't put a halt to all the uncomfortable symptoms that many women experience during menopause.

Some hang around for the rest of your days, and others may ease up over time:

- Less lubrication in the vagina
- Easy weight gain (and a harder time getting those extra pounds/kilos off!)
- Less control over your bladder and potential to get urinary tract infections (this goes with a newly developed ability to find the nearest public loo!)
- Poor sleep, or at least fewer really good nights than before
- Loss of bone mass – potential for osteoporosis
- Potential to develop high blood pressure, heart disease
- Even the occasional hot flush, and
- Possible periods of 'fuzzy' thinking and poor memory.

For most women, however, these are more than compensated for by a wonderful sense of well-being.

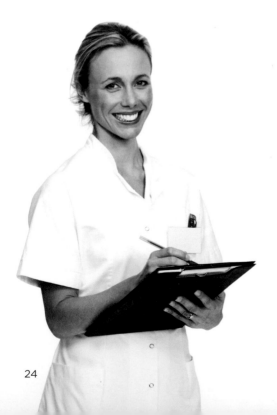

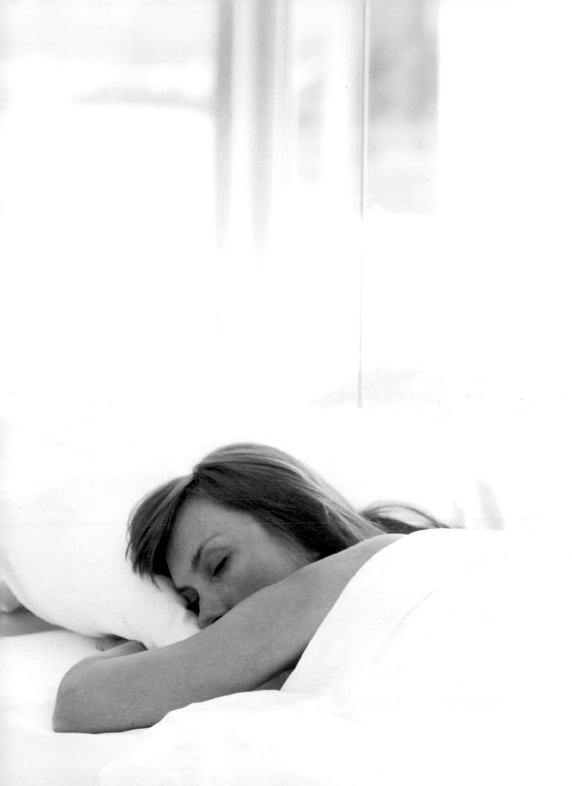

Q 29: I overheard some women using the term 'medical menopause'. Can you please explain what this is?

The terms medical menopause and surgical menopause sometimes get mixed up, so I'll deal with both in answer to your question.

Surgical menopause occurs when a woman has to undergo some type of surgery that removes her ovaries, or, as in the case of a full hysterectomy, her uterus along with the ovaries. When that happens, not only does she cease to be fertile, but her oestrogen levels drop dramatically.

Medical menopause also refers to circumstances where a woman experiences the same dramatic fall in oestrogen levels, though in some circumstances this may not be permanent. What happens in medical menopause is that some sort of medical intervention – chemotherapy, for example, pelvic radiation treatment or some therapies used to suppress oestrogen production for treatment reasons – causes damage to a woman's ovaries or suppresses her ability to produce oestrogen and progesterone.

For women who lose their ovaries or ovarian function through either surgical or medical intervention, menopause will arrive abruptly. This can make life particularly difficult, particularly for women only in their twenties and thirties, as they will most likely find themselves with all the symptoms of menopause.

Hormone therapy to replace what their bodies can no longer produce seems to be the answer here for most women, either as oestrogen alone or in combination with progestin. Best advice, of course, is that if you find yourself facing either form of forced menopause, make sure you ask your medical practitioner all the questions you can think of before treatment begins.

Women whose ovaries stay intact after surgery or treatment usually find they experience a normal transition to menopause.

Q 30: I have a friend who's considering having a hysterectomy because her family history with menopause is so bad and she doesn't want to go through it. Is this a good option?

The short answer is 'No' because a hysterectomy will stop the bleeding but do nothing for any of the other symptoms of menopause.

In our mothers' and grandmothers' day, hysterectomies were a lot more common than they are now. Nowadays they are only recommended for compelling medical reasons, despite the fact keyhole surgery techniques make them much less invasive than they used to be.

According to the Australian Institute of Health and Welfare, the number of hysterectomies performed in Australia has dropped by 58 per cent in just the last two decades, and numbers are similar in other advanced countries.

Some women, however, are looking to take control of their bleeding at the time of menopause by seeking elective hysterectomy. They then follow this with an ongoing regime of hormone replacement.

That's one way of doing it, but it's a big call. Hysterectomy is major surgery and so cannot be risk-free. The statistics point to the fact one woman in 1000 will face life-threatening complications or death from having a hysterectomy.

We used to say the same thing about childbirth by caesarean, but now many women are opting for it by choice, so they have a sense of control over their lives and bodies. Perhaps, in the same way, in some 20 years' time we'll wonder what all the fuss about choosing hysterectomy to circumvent menopause was for.

But, like all things in life, each woman to their own choices ...

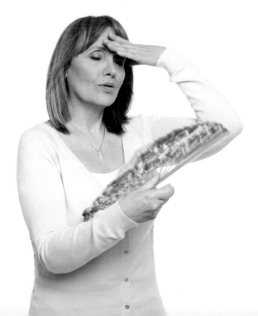

Women sum up their experience ...

"I noticed my behaviour changing, but I didn't know why. Naming it as the beginning of menopause really helped me feel that I had some control back."

"I am in my mid-40s. My periods have become irregular for the last four or five months and I was suffering from quite severe depression. I went to my doctor and asked if it could be menopause. He said 'You just need more exercise.' I went through a period of great uncertainty, not knowing if I was falling apart."

"I found the hot flushes the hardest thing to deal with. I would be looking around to see if anyone else was hot and then realise it was just me. Then I would try and act as if everything was normal."

"I found at work, under pressure, the hot flushes would come on."

"I would wake in the middle of the night. I would find this time my blackest time. I would feel really alone."[4]

Managing Menopause – the traditional Western medicine way

What's new?

- Hormone therapy (HT) now has the experts' tick of approval. Using HT to manage the symptoms of menopause and beyond is safe, according to the 2012 findings of an international group of organisations working on women's health and menopause issues. Their *Global Consensus Statement on Menopausal Hormone Therapy* claims the benefits of taking HT outweigh any negatives for women under 60.
- If you're over 60, however, or 10 years from menopause, be cautious and seek good advice. Long-term and making a late start on HT have been linked to a slight increase in breast cancer risk.
- Internationally renowned endocrinologist and menopause specialist, Professor Henry Burger, advises that HT is best used in the lead-up to the last period if symptoms are bothersome and as long as they remain so. HT is also appropriate where bone loss is a major problem.
- Taking HT cannot be a 'one size fits all' process, but needs to be individualised to suit each woman's specific needs.
- And, having said all that, the jury is still out, and much of the research is contradictory. The findings of another study released tomorrow or the day after might well come up with entirely different results again.
- So the recommendation really has to be – take the lowest dose possible of any prescribed medications and for as long as required to relieve symptoms or protect bones, providing the benefits and risks are clearly understood.

I know I'm repeating myself, but menopause is just another stage of life for most healthy women, and how a woman manages the transition is one more facet in the complex matrix of demands that comprises life for most women in the Western world.

Because it's a normal part of life, menopause does not require medicating, except where its symptoms make life unpleasant or intolerable. For those women there is help in the form of various hormone replacement therapies. Some other women choose to medicate for lifestyle and convenience issues, rather than a medical response to symptoms – and there's nothing wrong with that, either.

Apart from medical/pharmaceutical options, various natural alternative treatments are available. We'll look at these a little later in this book.

Menopause is not without its politics, however, with proponents of so-called natural hormones fiercely opposed to the use of what they see as synthetic alternatives. We'll cover some of this debate in the next section on bioidentical hormones.

Now, let's look at the more traditional approach still favoured by the majority of medical practitioners in the UK and Australia, and, perhaps to a lesser extent, in the USA.

Q 31: What are my medical options when menopausal symptoms make life miserable?

The first step is to see your medical practitioner. The first sign your periods are becoming irregular indicates it's time for a check-up; it is important to know that the change is due to perimenopause and is not a sign of any other medical condition.

If your symptoms are making life miserable, then the most obvious medical option is some form of Hormone Therapy (HT). HT is a general term for hormones prescribed to balance/replace the levels of a woman's natural hormones as her own hormone production fluctuates/declines before and after menopause.

The main hormones involved are oestrogen and progesterone, and in some cases, testosterone.

The best known HT is Hormone Replacement Therapy (HRT). These days HRT is also simply referred to as Hormone Therapy. This is in order to avoid the misleading message that HRT's purpose is to replace a woman's own hormones on an on-going basis. Though some women do choose to continue HT for many years after menopause, enabling them to maintain pre-menopausal hormone levels into later life, this is not the foremost purpose of HT.

In this book, we're using the letters HT.

HT comes in several forms, including:

- The most common form, containing oestrogen and progestin.
- The birth control pill, which also contains both oestrogen and progestin. These can be used before menopause both to treat perimenopausal symptoms and prevent pregnancy.
- Progestin-only pills, which can be used in a cyclical fashion to treat heavy menstrual bleeding associated with perimenopause.
- Oestrogen replacement therapy (ERT), or oestrogen-only HT. This is generally used by women who have had hysterectomies (had their uterus removed).
- Tibolone, which is converted in the body to oestrogenic, progestogenic and androgenic substances and is like conventional HT.

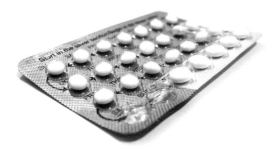

Q 32: Are other medical treatments also prescribed?

Other medications that may be prescribed include:

- Low-dose antidepressants. For women who can't take oestrogen, a low dose antidepressant that's part of the broad selective serotonin reuptake inhibitors (SSRIs) family of drugs is sometimes prescribed to help control hot flushes. It is also used for menopausal-type mood disorders.
- A drug that is used to treat seizures – Gabapentin (Neurontin) – is sometimes prescribed for reducing hot flushes.
- A blood pressure medication may also be used to control flushes (Clonidine or Catapres).

Q 33: Is it easy to get a prescription for HT?

Prior to prescribing HT, your medical practitioner will usually take a full family history and organise a range of examinations and tests. These are likely to include a pelvic and breast examination, blood tests for liver function, blood sugar, cholesterol, thyroid function, triglycerides, and calcium, phosphorus and iron levels.

You may also find yourself undergoing a bone density scan to check whether you may be particularly at risk of developing osteoporosis (bone loss), always a danger for post-menopausal women.

Q 34: When is HT prescribed – for the time leading up to menopause or for the time afterwards, or for both? And how long should I be on it?

Professor Burger advises that HT is best taken both before and after menstruation stops, as symptoms require.

He suggests women consider using hormone treatment when hot flushes and other symptoms are causing genuine inconvenience to their lives. He says if this is going to happen, it usually occurs in the year or so leading up to the last period and for approximately two or so years afterwards.

"Some women find that hot flushes return out of the blue some years later, for no apparent reason. At this stage, we don't know why it happens," Professor Burger says. "Women in their sixties, seventies and beyond sometimes find themselves having the odd hot flush.

"My advice to these women is to try a very low dose hormone patch until the flushes settle down again, as they usually do fairly quickly."

Q 35: What about long term HT use?

As far as Professor Burger is concerned, he recommends women take HT as long as required except in one particular circumstance – and that is where women suffer major bone loss and are in danger of fractures, where it should be given for at least five years, providing benefit and risk are clearly understood.

The reason is that taking HT for a long time slightly raises a woman's risk of developing breast cancer.

Professor Burger's confidence in HT use is generally in line with the findings of a group of international women's health organisations, which published guidelines for menopausal HT use early in 2013.

The *Global Consensus Statement on Menopausal Hormone Therapy* concludes:

- HT (or Menopausal Hormone Therapy – MHT, as it is referred to in the statement) is the most effective treatment for symptom related to the hormonal changes of menopause, such as hot flushes and sleep deprivation. MHT is also beneficial for bone health and may decrease mortality and cardiovascular disease.
- Risks associated with MHT are acknowledged, but benefits derived from MHT will generally outweigh the risks for women under 60, or within 10 years of the menopause. The risks are generally small.
- Taking MHT is a decision which needs to be individualised, according to a woman's symptoms, and her individual health status (such as age, time since menopause, family history, general health, has she had a hysterectomy or not, and other personal risk factors). This decision should be taken in consultation with a suitably qualified physician.

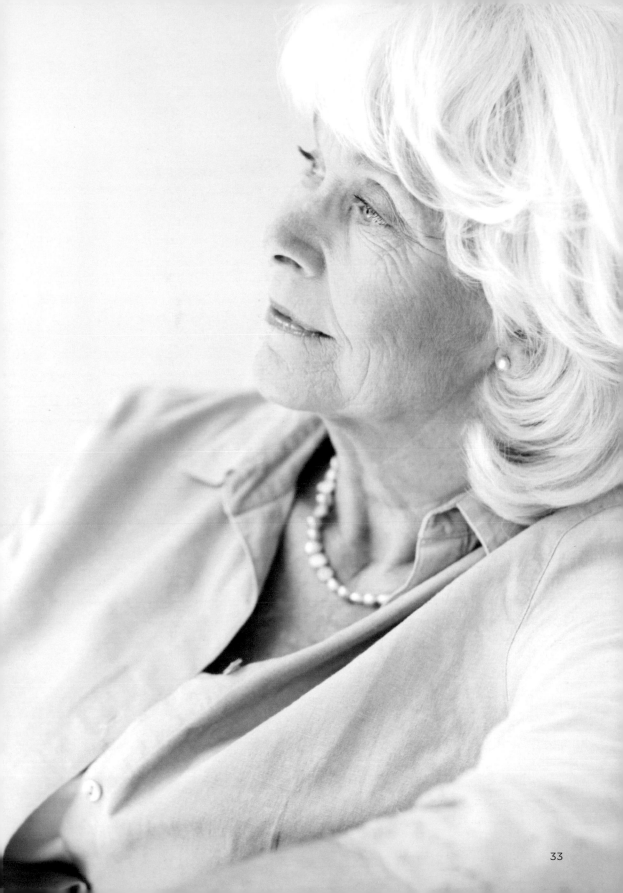

That is, the health organisations recommend women do not use HT post-menopause, for protection against heart disease, cancer and dementia. The Task Group panel assessed the findings from research around the world, and concluded the risks of long-term HT use for disease prevention outweighed its potential benefits.

One woman's hot flush surprise!

"I am now in my late sixties and reached menopause a decade or more ago – but three times lately I've suddenly found myself having a hot flush. At first I thought it must have been something else, that I must have been sickening for something – but no, these were classic, if mild, hot flushes.

"I never realised women could still get them, both at my age and so long after menopause, but when I did some online research I realised I'm not alone; it's quite common for the odd hot flush to catch even women in the seventies and eighties by surprise!

"At least it was mild, so that's a blessing. I don't want to go through that whole menopause process again."
Cheryl-Ann P, Williamsburg, USA

Q 36: If I go down the HT track, what's it going to do for me?

We've gone through all the symptoms of perimenopause, and HT will help with most of these, e.g. dry vagina, hot flushes, night sweats, aches and pains etc, and even mood swings.

There are some other benefits that replacing hormones using HT may bring, though these are not yet fully understood. Here replacing oestrogen seems to be the key to, in some measure at least:
• Preventing osteoporosis developing or at least delaying its onset
• Possibly delaying the onset of Alzheimer's disease
• Reducing cholesterol levels
• And possibly helping prevent or delay the development of colon cancer and age-related eye-disease (macular degeneration).

And then there's the fact that many women claim it improves the quality of their skin and hair and makes them look and feel younger. And who can argue with that?

Q 37: What happens when I stop taking HT?

After you've been taking HT for some time, perhaps two years or so, your medical practitioner will usually recommend you give the medication a short break to see if you still need it. If menopausal symptoms return, then it's probably not time to stop using HT yet. If they don't then you can probably say your time of needing this help to get through menopause is over.

Some women can stop using HT 'cold turkey', that is, stop one day and have no adverse effects whatsoever, and no return of hot flushes etc.

Others find they do much better if they wean themselves off the hormones gradually. Even if they're past menopause, withdrawing from the replacement hormones can be as severe as the symptoms of menopause itself. The general advice from medical practitioners is that a slow reduction in dosages over a period of months is best.

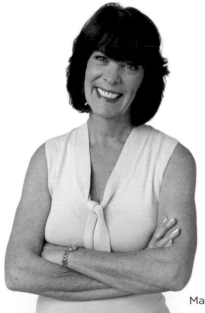

June's story

"When I went onto HT it was like a miracle and I felt like a new woman. My libido came back and I was energised at work again ... life was good.

"I stayed on it for five years and then had to switch doctors because I moved to another city. My new one did not like women to be on hormone replacement long term, so I stopped taking it. It was hell; it was like all those symptoms I had avoided over the past five years – the hot flushes and crabbiness, the loss of libido, energy and enthusiasm for life, the night sweats – had just been waiting in the background to take their revenge on me! I thought I was going to die. But I chose not to go back onto HT, but just to live through it. Which I did, and now life is great. But when I think about it now, I should have gradually reduced the dose I took, so my body could adjust slowly."
June T, Canberra, Australia

Q 38: When did women first start using HRT, can you let me know a bit about its history?

Even though our mothers probably didn't take hormones back in their day, assisting women with menopause symptoms by replacing oestrogen isn't new. Oestrogen and progesterone were first isolated in USA laboratories in the 1920s, though their use was primarily for women who had gone through a surgical menopause for some reason or another, or who suffered from severe menstrual cramps.

The first brand of HT used extensively in the USA became available in 1942 and was prescribed mainly for its capacity to keep women 'youthful'. It contained oestrogens isolated from pregnant mares' urine which, when absorbed into the blood, convert to oestradiol, an active oestrogen found in women. This type of oestrogen is known as conjugated equine oestrogen, and is still one of the products used in HT today.

By the 1950s, HT was being widely prescribed to American women for treating perimenopausal symptoms and for enhancing youthfulness and appearance after menopause, but some concerns were raised about an otherwise unexplained rise in the incidence of cancer of the uterus lining. By the mid-1970s use of HT had declined rapidly and remained at low levels for some years until forms of the medication combining oestrogen with progestins proved to eliminate the uterine cancer risk.

Some definitions

Progesterone is a hormone naturally produced in the body and plays a significant role in enabling a woman to maintain a pregnancy.

Progestin is the name of synthetically-manufactured progesterone. Both natural and synthetically produced progesterones are known collectively as progestogens.

By the late 1990s, however, many women had started questioning their medical practitioners' ready prescription of HT at the first sign of menopausal symptoms.

Q 39: Was the women's concern justified?

These concerns seemed to be confirmed when a long-term trial of HRT by the Women's Health Initiative (WHI) was stopped in 2002, three years short of its scheduled completion date because results linked HT use with various health risks.

This WHI study was conducted under the auspice of the US National Heart, Lung, and Blood Institute (NHLBI), part of the US National Institutes of Health (NIH).

The WHI undertook clinical trials and observational research over 15 years with more than 160,000 postmenopausal women aged between 50 and 79. Primary research foci were cardiovascular disease, cancer and osteoporosis, and women were followed, on average for just over five years.

The trial was stopped for the 160,000 women who were included in the HRT part of the research project when findings indicated women using both forms of HT – oestrogen-progestin and oestrogen alone – increased their risk of suffering stroke and blood clots. The results also showed women taking the combined medication also increased their risk of suffering heart attack and breast cancer.

There was some good news in the study findings – both forms of HT reduced the number of hip and other fractures they were likely to suffer, while those on the combined hormone treatment had a decreased risk of experiencing colorectal cancer.

The publication of WHI research results and subsequent publicity sent shock waves around the world, with women in the millions deciding to quit taking HT there and then.

Q 40: What happened next?

According to Professor Burger, women suffered unnecessarily because a decade on from the release of the WHI study findings, medical professionals have concluded its conclusions were flawed. HT is now considered safe for the majority of women who need it.

Professor Burger estimates that in the aftermath of the fear and anxiety releasing the study result caused, some 80 per cent of women in the USA stopped using any form of hormone therapy, as did some 50 per cent of Australian women.

"Perhaps half these women saw a sudden return to their symptoms and their quality of life suffered accordingly," Professor Burger says.

Q 41: What does the latest research say?

Two subsequent substantial reviews of the evidence have pointed to flaws in the WHI study.

Professor Burger says these flaws include:
- Women in the study had an average age of 63, so were not the usual group prescribed HT.
- The findings confused 'relative risk' and 'absolute risk', leading to the conclusion the risk for women of getting breast cancer, for example, was 26 per cent higher for women on HT than for those who did not take it. In fact, the 'actual risk' increases by only one tenth of one per cent (from about three per 1000 per year to just under four per 1000 per year).
- The increased risk of heart disease found in the study was age-related, and occurred primarily in the 21 per cent of women in the study who were 70-79 years old at the start.

Professor Burger says healthy women who use HT around the time of menopause do not increase their risk of heart disease, and it is safe and effective for women who suffer from hot flushes, poor sleep patterns and night sweats, either around the time of menopause or in the five-10 years.

He points to other advantages of its use, as well as its role in maintaining bone density. For example, it almost certainly reduces the risk of heart disease, diabetes and colorectal cancer and may play a role in reducing the risk of dementia. Overall, it generally improves quality of life for menopausal women as well.

Q 42: HT usually comes as a tablet, but I hate swallowing pills; is there another way to take it?

HT is available in tablet form, but there are other options, for example, skin patches, skin gel, implants and vaginal preparations such as creams or tablets.

Some women may need to try out several methods of delivery before they find the one that suits them best, and this process may take several months.

Let's go through the options:
- Different kinds of tablets - Oestrogen and progesterone can be taken separately or as combined tablets. They come in packs like the contraceptive pill so it's easy to check whether you've taken your dose or not. Dosages and types vary.
- Patches - Patches ensure the hormones are absorbed directly through the skin into the blood stream. Some patches contain oestrogen while others provide a combination of both oestrogen and progesterone. Patch size varies according to hormone dosage.
- As a gel, which comes in single dose sachets and is rubbed into the skin, usually daily.
- Creams and pessaries – these are inserted directly into the vagina. These are usually prescribed when a woman and her partner are troubled by perhaps the most unwelcome outcomes of menopause – vaginal dryness and bladder problems.
- As implants, which are inserted under the skin.

Progestin on its own may come as a tablet, a patch or an intrauterine device or IUD. Testosterone, which is usually only prescribed short-term, comes in the form of a cream or an implanted slow-release pellet. It's mainly used to deal with libido issues.

You should find, if your medical practitioner is on the ball, he or she will start you on a low dose whatever the chosen medication and review your progress often.

and though the risk is low, for vulnerable women it can be life-threatening.

As we've seen in the research, long-term HRT use does increase the risk of breast cancer slightly (three women in 1000 per year to four women in 1000).

And occasionally a woman will experience break-through bleeding, but again, this may simply require a change of dosage or brand.

Q 43: I've heard women complain about side effects of taking HT? Are there any and, if so, what are they?

Some women complain that it makes them feel sick, others that they feel bloated and that fluid builds up around their ankles or even faces. Others claim it makes their breasts feel sore, that they get leg cramps when they never had them before, and that it's the cause of them feeling irritable a lot of the time, if not sometimes downright depressed.

If you can lay claim to any of the reactions I've listed, it's worth talking to your medical practitioner about changing the dosage you're taking, or perhaps swapping HT brands.

While these side effects can make life miserable, some others occur occasionally that can be much more serious. For example, some women on oestrogen pills (but not on patches) are at risk of developing blood clots (venous thrombosis),

Q 44: My mother suffered from high blood pressure and had a heart attack, does that rule me out from using HRT if I need it?

A: That's only something your medical practitioner can answer. He or she will look at your paternal history, not just your maternal, but I would say be very careful, and make sure you have all the appropriate pre-testing before you make up your mind.

A family history is certainly not a contra-indication to HT, but it may be preferable to using an oestrogen patch.

Q 45: In my early twenties, when I went on the contraceptive pill, I developed a varicose vein and was told to stop taking it. I developed several more when I was pregnant. Does this preclude me from using HT?

A: Again, this is an answer your medical practitioner is probably best qualified to provide, but you may like to consider using an oestrogen patch rather than HT in tablet form, as patches do not increase clotting risk.

Q 46: Would you please list what sort of health history might put me at risk if I opt to start HT?

A: Put simply, women in the 'at risk' category have:

- A history of breast cancer, personally or in the family
- Unexplained vaginal bleeding
- Other blood clotting disorders
- Some types of uterine (endometrial) cancer, and
- A range of other problems, including epilepsy, liver disease, migraine headaches, gall bladder disease and high blood pressure.

Putting your hand up for any of these doesn't necessarily mean you can't take HT, but it does mean be cautious.

A study reported in the Canadian Medical Association Journal in January 2014, claims post-menopausal use of HT may increase a woman's risk of acute pancreatitis or sudden onset of inflammation of the pancreas.

The study, conducted between 1997 and 2010, involved more than 31,000 Swedish women, all post menopausal and aged 48 at the start of the study. Just over 42 per cent were using some form of HT, 12 per cent had been previous users, and the remainder had never used it.

The study showed a small (1.5 per cent) increased risk of acute pancreatitis in women using HT, with the risk seeming greater in those who had taken it for at least a decade.

Oskarsson V, Orsini N, Sadr-Azodi O, Wolk A, *Postmenopausal hormone replacement therapy and risk of acute pancreatitis: a prospective cohort study*, CMAJ, 2014

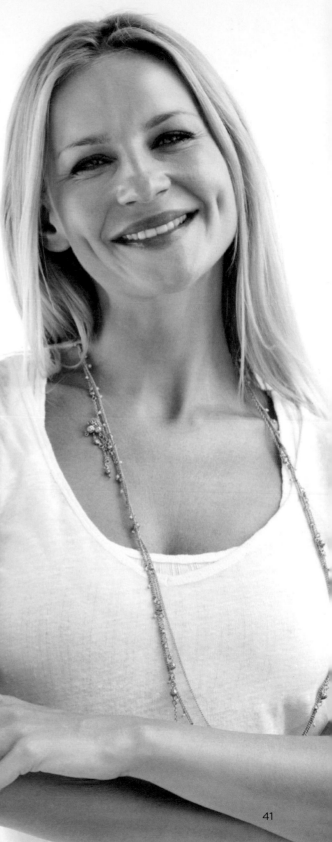

Q 47: What about women who reach menopause early? Should they take HT?

Women who have stopped having periods before 40, or have naturally (not surgically) lost normal ovary function before then are strongly recommended to consider taking HT of some description until the normal age of menopause.

If they leave starting it until they are 45, then they will be at a higher risk of developing a whole range of problems including coronary heart disease, osteoporosis, dementia, anxiety, depression and problems with their sexuality.

There is an upside, however, and that is women who reach menopause early have a lower risk of most breast and ovarian cancers than their sisters who reach it within the normal age range.

Q 48: Can I take HT to 'stop the clock'?

I hate how, now I'm past menopause, I'm starting to look so much older on the outside than I feel inside.

Like many questions around HT, the jury is out on this question.

Women on HT by-and-large claim to feel better on it, are generally happier, feel younger and more vital and are generally more content with life. They also ascribe having better concentration and memory as well as increased libido to taking the hormones.

Proponents claim HT has an anti-ageing effect on muscle and skin, with the hormones preventing skin thinning and sagging, particularly around the neck and jaw. It also helps women maintain good muscle tone throughout the whole body.

According to Professor Burger, there's only one genuine reason for taking HT apart from dealing with menopausal symptoms, and that's for women who have lost bone density and are in significant danger of bone fractures.

So he doesn't recommend it as a 'stopping the clock' option.

Q 49: Are there other views?

Results from an international study, published in the British Medical Journal, claim that if a woman starts taking HT soon after menopause she does not increase her risk of developing cancer, stroke or thrombosis with longer term use.

This study, done over a decade with 1000 Danish women, did however indicate there's only a narrow window of opportunity for women to achieve the health effects using HT after menopause may bring.

Women in this timing window need to be under 60 or be less than 10 years past menopause, and need to keep taking the hormones for six years.

When it comes to our health, nothing is simple and nothing is black and white!

Odd Spot

According to the UK-based Women's Health Concern, there are many women who have been taking HT without problems for 20 or 30 years. So that 70-year-old with youthful skin and pert body may not owe it all to the cosmetic surgeon's knife, but to the HT pill package instead.

Q 50: So I guess it's all a matter of who you speak to?

The advice from Jean Hailes for Women's Health is as follows.

MYTH – HT is too dangerous to take – it causes breast cancer.

FACT – For otherwise healthy women, taking hormone replacement therapy (HT) for two to five years to relieve menopausal symptoms causes little if any increase in breast cancer risk.

ADVICE – If you're not taking HT during menopause, you have a three in 1000 chance of developing breast cancer in a given year. If you take HT for five years, that chance goes up slightly to just under four in 1000. Weigh this small risk against the benefits of HT, which can significantly improve women's quality of life and reduce risks of osteoporosis, diabetes and colon cancer. Take the lowest effective dose of HT for only as long as required by your symptoms, and regularly review your reasons to continue (or not) with your health practitioner. HT can be stopped at any time, after which any increase in breast cancer risk lessens over time and is lost within five years.[5]

Q 51: You've only talked hormone therapies, but is that the only sort of medical help the medical profession can offer for menopause symptoms?

As mentioned before, medical practitioners do have some options, such as:

- The high blood pressure medication called clonidine, which seems to have some effect on reducing hot flushes.
- A couple of anti-depressant drugs also seem to help some women. They are paroxetine and venlafaxine, and
- A medication for epilepsy and chronic pain management, called gabapentin, has also been shown to be effective where hot flushes are extreme.

Again, the advice is to see your clinician and ask your questions directly.

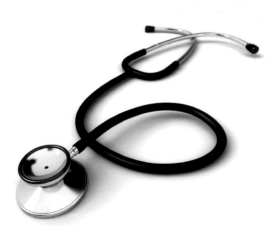

Bioidentical hormones – the case for and against

What's new?

- While women who use compounded bioidentical hormones swear by them, the jury is still out on their safety, and is likely to remain so until long-term trials have been undertaken.
- According to one expert, they have their place in the range of options available to women, but there's no good data supporting claims the bioidentical hormones are any different from traditional HT.
- Concerns remain that bioidentical hormones can be dispensed on the whim of a prescribing physician and compounding pharmacist, with no quality assurance.

Odd Spot

Women have used genuine bioidentical hormones for many thousands of years. History records that ageing Chinese noble women treated problems associated with menopause by eating the dried urine of young women, and that other women down the ages also resorted to this treatment regime. Young women's urine is rich in the metabolic waste products of the hormones that can cause menopausal women such grief as their levels decline – oestrogen, progesterone and testosterone.

Q 52: So what are bioidentical hormones and how do they differ from the hormones I take in my regular HT tablets?

Bioidentical hormone replacement therapy (BHRT) or bioidentical hormone therapy (BHT) are terms used to describe menopause medication where the replacement hormones are plant-sourced (phytoestrogens) and said to be identical on a molecular level to the chemicals produced by women's own bodies. Hence the term 'bioidentical'.

The hormones in question are oestrogen in various forms, progesterone and, at times, other hormones such as testosterone.

Proponents of BHT claim this form of hormone therapy, in contrast to normal HT, is 'natural', and so allows women to deal with menopause 'naturally'.

The traditional HT hormones, oestrogen and progestin, are synthesised from sources including the urine of pregnant mares; some are not molecularly the same as those found in the human body while others are. This is true especially of oestradiol in patches and progesterone as tablets, creams or suppositories, obtainable with some difficulty in Australia for HT.

In a world where more and more women are looking for holistic health solutions, this difference is seen as a marketing plus for bioidenticals; the 'natural' tag can be a great marketing tool for any product in a competitive market, and the market for hormone replacement products is definitely a competitive one.

For a woman the idea she can find relief from menopausal symptoms or even reverse the ageing process in a natural way, one that mimics the workings of her own body can be very persuasive.

The term 'natural' though, is always open to interpretation. Is using plant products as the basis for introduced hormones any more natural that using animal-derived products? That's a question that's not yet been properly answered, though strong advocates exist for both sides of the debate.

Q 53: Is BHT popular?

The market for BHT has been much stronger in the USA than it has been in either the UK or Australia, although its use is now increasing in the latter countries.

The scare caused in 2002 by the findings of the WHI research into HT, linking its use to increased risk of cancer, gave the BHT industry a great push along.

Though the use of custom-compounded BHRT was for some time restricted to the USA it is no longer, and more and more women in that country now use both the compounded and commercially-produced bioidentical preparations.

Q 54: What are compounded bioidentical hormones?

Compounded bioidentical hormones are prepared individually from, primarily, plant-based phytoestrogens. Their composition is worked out in accordance to a woman's individual hormone levels at the time those hormones levels are tested. So, a woman needs regular blood tests to assess hormone levels each time she has her prescription for compounded bioidentical hormone therapy filled out.

The word 'compounded' is used because this form of HT is prepared, or compounded, individually by chemists/pharmacists, rather than being produced en masse by pharmaceutical companies.

Some forms of bioidentical hormone products, produced by pharmaceutical companies, are available over-the-counter from drug stores, pharmacies and chemists. In Australia, for example, the appropriate government agency, the Therapeutic Goods Administration (TGA), has approved the use of oestradiol patches, which are sometimes referred to as 'bioidenticals' and are readily available, but has not approved compounded treatments.

In the United States the Food and Drug Administration (FDA) has given its okay to the use of bioidentical progesterone and oestrogen oestradiol, as produced by pharmaceutical companies in standard dosages, but has not approved the compounded version. Like non-bioidentical HT products, commercially produced BHT packages must carry appropriate warnings about potential risks of use.

Compounded BHT is not FDA-approved and so compounding pharmacies aren't required to provide clients with details of potential use risks.

Q 55: What's the case for BHT?

The arguments for and against using BHT are quite technical, but for our purposes we've summed them up simply.

The FOR case

According to the BHT industry:

1. Bioidentical hormones are identical to the hormone molecules produced naturally in the body.

Bioidentical hormones are synthesised from precursor molecules found in wild yams and soybeans and can be easily converted for human use.

2. BHT can be administered in ways that allow it to enter the blood stream directly, avoiding the digestive system and producing less stress on the liver. Methods include as a lozenge (troche), a cream rubbed onto the skin (a transdermal cream), patches and gels. It is these delivery systems which have been patented by pharmaceutical companies, not the hormone products themselves.

3. While some bioidentical hormone products can be bought over-the-counter, they can also be prepared individually – or custom compounded by compounding chemists/pharmacists. This means they are available to women in preparations that meet their individual needs, according to their own specific hormone levels.

4. Technically the body can't distinguish bioidentical hormones from the ones produced by a woman's ovaries. Therefore, proponents claim it's possible to monitor levels of oestrogen, for example, more accurately than with traditional HRT, and adjust treatment levels accordingly.

5. The US FDA has approved the use of some forms of bioidentical hormone therapy, though these are only available on prescription and not prepared individually.

One US woman swears she could not live without her compounded bioidentical hormone treatment

In her early sixties, Mary A takes BHT every day.

"If someone told me they were going to take my hormones therapy away, I'd be really angry. I intend to keep on taking them for years yet – for as long as I can. When I stopped for a little while a couple of years ago back came the hot flashes and I couldn't sleep at night because of the sweats.

The worst thing, however, was the depression that went with it. I just can't live with that. I tried taking the ordinary HT pill, but that didn't really do much for me. I'm sticking with bioidenticals from my compounding pharmacist because I know I'm getting the right dose of hormones for me, not just a general dose. I have regular blood tests to make sure my prescriptions meet my needs. So, please, don't talk to me about the case against bioidenticals; I just don't want to know."

Q 56: What's the case against BHT?

Despite recommendations like Mary A's, there is a case against bioidenticals, with regulating authorities yet to give the therapy a full tick of approval.

The AGAINST case

1. Bioidentical hormones are manufactured synthetically by a similar process to most hormones, including those used in the pill and traditional HT, hence using the term 'natural' is a misnomer. They are synthetically produced.

2. Custom compounding – that is making a woman's BHT dose specifically to match her own needs – makes it difficult for these medications to be approved by bodies such as the TGA and FDA because each woman's prescription will be unique. That means they miss out on testing that might prove whether the ingredients are absorbed appropriately or react how they are expected to in a woman's blood and body.

3. Assessing a woman's hormone levels through testing blood or saliva is a hit-and-miss process because those levels vary considerably throughout the day and from day to day during the midlife years.

4. There's limited quality control over the preparation of prescription BHT products by compounding chemists/pharmacists.

5. There is no published evidence that BHT from compounding pharmacists is safe to use and carries no health risks. As a form of hormone replacement, it carries the same possible health risks for women as other HT – e.g. blood clots, breast and uterine cancer, heart problems etc.

6. Long-term clinical trials have not been undertaken yet into the use of hormones from compounding pharmacies, so risks associated with their use, if any, aren't fully known. This concern is exacerbated by the fact that, in some instances, hormone doses in BHT are 10 times greater than doses of comparable HT products.

7. Compounding pharmacists, at least in the US, aren't required to report side effects from the bioidentical hormones they prepare and dispense.

The FDA claims blood and saliva tests are not useful in setting hormone doses for individual women. These tests, they say, indicate a woman's hormone levels at that one moment in time. It's not possible, however, to get accurate correlations between hormone levels in the saliva or blood levels and a woman's menopausal symptoms. That is, there's not a 'norm' when it comes to saliva and blood levels and an individual woman's symptoms. Each woman is different, so these tests cannot be a reliable indicator on which to base BHT preparation.

In summary

There is as yet no long-term, evidence-based research to test the safety and effectiveness of bioidentical hormone preparations, in particular those prepared by compounding chemists/pharmacists. The TGA and the FDA have not approved the use of compounded products and are unlikely to do so until they have access to the results of trials and quality published research.
In addition, some well-known organisations (e.g. International Menopause Society and the North American Menopause Society) have suggested risks associated with using BHT should be treated the same as the risks of using traditional HRT, until such time as their safety is proven by longitudinal trials.

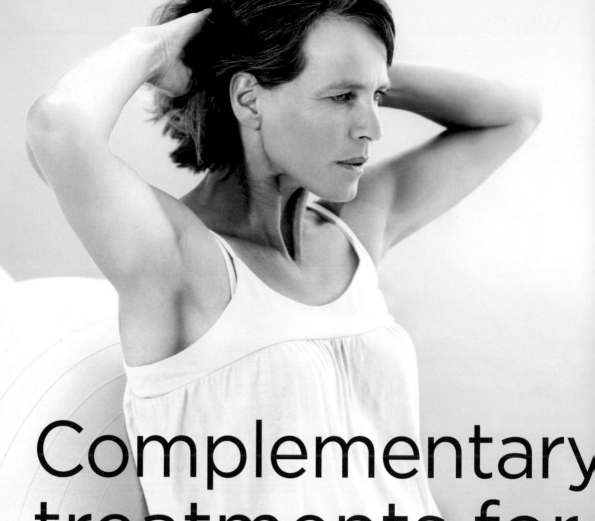

Complementary treatments for menopause symptoms

What's new?

- The either/or – Western medicine or natural alternatives – approach is giving way to one where all the disciplines of health care are considered to have a legitimate place in healing.
- Explore complementary treatments for yourself – but make sure you do it with the advice of properly qualified practitioners.
- The herb black cohosh, linked to several liver damage cases in Australia, has now been given a tick as safe to use. Some small concerns remain and the advice is to restrict use to no more than six months continuously.[6]

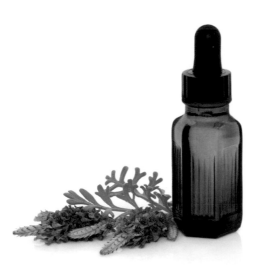

Q 57: If bioidentical hormone treatment is the newest thing in medical treatment, is there anything new in the complementary medicine?

Many women prefer to turn to alternative or complementary therapies to ease their way through menopause rather than take the medical route.

They view complementary treatments as a gentler way to handle their symptoms and consider something that can be tagged 'natural' more likely to be healthier and have fewer side effects than its medical counterparts.

The either/or – Western medicine or natural alternatives – approach is giving way to one where all the disciplines of health care are considered legitimate and the aim is to have them working together to provide the best and most non-intrusive menopause transition possible. So, in essence, the term 'complementary medicine' implies any of the healthcare disciplines, including Western medicine, can be used together to prevent and manage health complaints.

Q 58: I notice you're using the word 'complementary'; isn't the usual word 'alternative'?

Traditional health and complementary health practitioners now prefer to use the word 'complementary' rather than 'alternative' when referring to non-pharmaceutical menopause therapies, as the preferred word reflects a shift to a more inclusive attitude and approach to treatment.

A 2007 UK study[7] into women's attitudes to menopause treatments found 95 per cent of respondents said they would try complementary therapies before HT in the belief they were more natural, and more than two-thirds (68 per cent) were prepared to pay considerably more for such treatment than the costs of HT. The study also found 73 per cent of respondents said they did not know enough about HT to make an informed choice.

Q 59: Is complementary medicine popular?

Complementary medicine is already used widely in Western countries. In Australia, for example, the National Institute of Complementary Medicine (NICM) reported in August 2010 that two in three Australians had used complementary medicines in the previous 12 months.

This amounted to a more-than A$3.5 billion spend on complementary therapies and medicines, with many of the chosen interventions aimed at managing chronic diseases such as osteoarthritis, and so improving quality of life.

Q 60: So, what are you actually talking about when you use the term 'complementary' therapies?

The underlying principle of complementary medicines and therapies is that the body can heal itself with a little help. This goes hand-in-hand with the idea that prevention is easier and better than cure.

For simplicity's sake, we'll use the letters CT to refer to everything that comes under the complementary medicine/therapy umbrella.

The field of CT is wide indeed. It covers everything from specific therapeutic practices such as naturopathy, acupuncture and homeopathy to body and energy work therapies and practices such as massage, tai chi, yoga and the energy release methods of Network Care or Network Spinal Analysis. This latter therapy originally developed out of chiropractic. The complementary field also includes nutrition, herbs and Chinese medicines, and methods of working with the breath, and much more.

Some of these therapies have been available to menopausal women since time immemorial, while others are still in their infancy. Network Care is one of the latter, as is the paced respiration method advocated by, amongst others, Professor Robert Freedman of the School of Medicine at Wayne State University in Detroit, USA.

Q 61: I know that HT works when it comes to menopausal symptoms, but how do some of these other therapies work?

I don't think I can answer that question; all I can do is go through some therapies and treatments in a little detail.

Let's start with **naturopathy**, which is probably the best known of these complementary therapies.

Naturopathy has a proud history, having its roots back in the healing traditions that have evolved from ancient Europe. Picture, if you will, the wise women of older societies we've probably all read about, collecting their herbs and compounding their treatments; these women, and men too of course, were the forerunners of today's naturopaths.

Naturopathy defines health as a positive state of physical and mental wellness and it works on the idea that the body can heal itself, given the right conditions and assistance. Rather than disease being diagnosed at the end stage, *illness is* detected at the earliest stage by looking

for risk factors, examining the diet for deficiencies and working out what needs to be changed to help the functioning of the body.

Q 62: What does treatment involve?

Treatment is provided whether the disease is chronic (i.e. longer term and on-going) or acute and usually combines nutrition, diet, lifestyle and the provision of appropriate herbal medicine.

For women going through menopause, a naturopath has the option of choosing from a wide variety of herbs and supplements.

These might include nutritional supplements such as calcium and magnesium, vitamins D and E, and the essential fatty acids omega-3, 6 and 9, plus a variety of herbal remedies. Some, such as black cohosh and shatavari (the root of a type of asparagus plant from India), red clover, wild yam and lady's mantle are said to help adjust hormonal imbalances in women. Licorice root is also said to be effective.

NOTE
Before you go ahead and raid the supplement shelves of the health store, please check with a naturopath, your medical practitioner or other therapist well versed in the use of supplements etc. You need to know that what you're taking is right for you. This warning is particularly important if you happen to be taking any other forms of medication or supplements.

Q 63: How does this compare with Chinese Medicine?

Chinese Medicine has its own specific theory about menopause.

The traditional wisdom of the discipline claims menopause takes place when a woman's body starts to preserve blood and energy in order to maintain her vitality and the nourishment of the various organs of the body, especially the kidneys. The kidneys are the organs, according to Chinese Medicine, that are the root of life and vitality.

Chinese Medicine believes the body has its own wisdom, and menopause is part of this process. Menopause is a process of transition, moving women through a real 'change of life' – from the mother stage to the stage of being an enlightened and wise being.

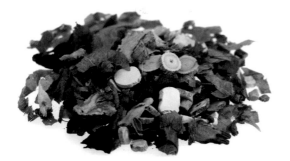

Author's indulgence

I guess I don't have to reiterate what I said in my introduction – that my own experience of living through the years of menopause and a decade or more since is that the Chinese have it right; the years post-menopause can be the best and freest of life. I personally would not swap this stage the Chinese maintain is dedicated to enlightenment and wisdom for anything. Mind you, I'm not claiming to be wise or enlightened, just content with being free to be who I am!

Chinese Medicine proponents claim a combination of acupuncture and Chinese herbal medicine can detect energy changes happening in a woman's body in perimenopause. Treatments can then be designed to relieve symptoms such as hot flushes, mood swings and the sense many women have that they've lost their capacity to think clearly. They can back up the effectiveness of such treatment with evidence from medical literature that goes back to the time of Jesus Christ!

While you'll need to see a proper Chinese Medicine practitioner rather than dabble yourself, one naturopath I spoke to recommended people plagued by menopausal insomnia check out the Chinese herb zizyphus.

Q 64: How does homeopathy differ from naturopathy and Chinese Medicine?

Homeopathy is less well understood and accepted than naturopathy or Chinese Medicine. It originated in Europe in the late 18th Century and is based on the principle that 'like cures like'. The therapy's name reflects this principle, coming from two Greek words meaning 'like' and 'suffering'.

A homeopath will treat a person with specially prepared, highly dilute preparations designed to stimulate a healing response and strengthen the body's ability to heal itself. The practitioner will assess all of the person's symptoms, mental and emotional as well as physical, and identify a remedy capable of producing in a healthy person's symptoms most 'like' the symptoms the person they're treating is suffering from. This helps the body come to its own healing.

Explained this way, homeopathy sounds counter-intuitive, which is why many proponents of traditional Western medicine find it hard to take seriously. But it has a long history of success stories and fans all over the world (of which I have to admit to being one).

My own homeopathic success story (one of many I am pleased to say!)

Many in the medical and scientific communities consider homeopathy to be not only ineffective but implausible as well, and they support this view with the findings of various research studies. I confess though that I'm a great advocate for it, and admit to being biassed; I have used homeopathy for many years and swear by it.

In fact, I regularly head for the homeopath before I head for the doctor, but only because I have proven in practice time and again how effective homeopathy has been for me. So, let me tell you my menopause story where homeopathy saved me from going under the knife – and scoff at it if you will.

I had an easy time going through perimenopause, with few hot flushes and those very mild, and my sleep disturbed some nights, but nothing much to bother about. Late in the process, however, I

found myself bleeding robustly for days/weeks on end. I went to my local medical practitioner who sent me for a scan, which indicated I had a huge benign cyst on one ovary. The medical solution? A hysterectomy and my life on hold for several weeks while I recovered.

I went to my homeopath before doing anything else. Diagnosis? Part of the pituitary gland, one of the master glands governing the functioning of the body's entire hormone system, was not functioning as effectively as it could. That was creating the hormone imbalance responsible for both the bleeding and the cyst. The solution? To get the pituitary working properly again.

I went home with my tiny bottle of homeopathic drops and by the end of the following day the bleeding had stopped. When my doctor ordered a second scan a few days later, the cyst had all but disappeared.

So, I'm a fan of homeopathy, no matter what the research might say. (Your homeopathy-hooked author.)

Q 65: You mentioned acupuncture as well. How does that work for menopause?

Acupuncture is a key component of traditional Chinese medicine and is among the oldest healing practices in the world. It involves various procedures that work on specific points in the body, with the aim of correcting imbalances in energy flows throughout the whole body.

Usually special needles are used to penetrate the skin at various points on the meridians or energy channels of the body, and these needles are then manipulated or stimulated electrically. While many in the Western scientific world still doubt the existence of these energy meridians, acupuncture has its firm fans and is growing rapidly in popularity in the USA, UK and Australia.

NOTE
The United Nations World Health Organisation has approved acupuncture as a treatment for menopausal symptoms and several studies are currently being conducted in USA, UK and Australia to see if this assessment is genuinely backed up in practice. For example, Australia's Melbourne University is currently running a major trial, in conjunction with Jean Hailes for Women's Health to test whether hot flushes can be tamed by acupuncture and be a suitable replacement for HRT for some women. While the trial is not complete, results so far indicate that it does work for some women, reducing the number and severity of hot flushes they experience, but is not effective in all cases.

One of the theories being considered is that acupuncture can be effective because it increases the serotonin levels in the body. Serotonin is the body's 'feel good' hormone. A two-year study at the University of Pittsburgh, USA, in the late 1990s showed acupuncture was effective in both reducing hot flushes (35 per cent decrease) and in improving sleep (50 per cent decrease in insomnia). It also showed those who continued with acupuncture treatment after the completion of the trial showed a significant decrease in the number of hot flushes they were experiencing post-menopause.

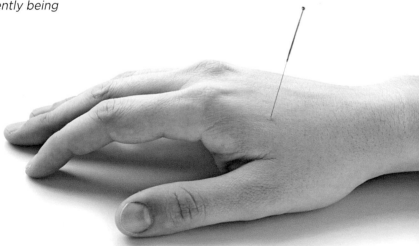

Q 66: Are there other complementary therapies worth trying?

Several manipulative therapies also fall under the complementary therapy tag. They may improve women's experience through menopause because they serve to release blockages and tensions in the body and so help it function better. This obviously promotes better general health and well-being. And for some menopausal women, that's enough.

These therapies – physiotherapy, osteopathy and chiropractic, for example – are based on the science of human mechanics, that is, how the body is structured and moves. Physiotherapy and chiropractic work strongly with the structure of the spine, while osteopathy's focus is on the way soft tissue affects the skeleton. All three, of course, aim to improve the body's general health through releasing pressures and tensions within the body's bone structure.

The *Alexander Technique* also works on the body. It provides a series of treatments and exercises that aim to change habits in the way we move that create problems within the body. In that way, it aims to re-educate both mind and body.

Q 67: You mentioned Network Care before, what is it?

Network Care, which you might also find under the trademarked name of Network Spinal Analysis, also works on re-educating the mind and body. It is an evidenced based approach to wellness and body awareness that had been developed over the past three decades by American chiropractor, Dr Donald Epstein.

It involves gentle touch on the spine, the aim of which is to improve the body's capacity to release tension and tap into its own self-healing capacities.

If what I have written above sounds like jargon, I apologise. I am a great fan of Network Care (and indeed of most complementary approaches to healing) and find it impossible to describe how it works, so all I can say is I know that it does work, or at least that it has worked for me.

Q 68: What are the herbal remedies recommended for menopause symptoms?

This is a question best answered by a naturopath or Chinese Medicine practitioner, but there are some herbal products readily available over the supermarket or health food store counter that work for some women.

Herbal remedies are favoured over pharmaceutical products by many women who see them being more gentle and natural. The downside is that their effects may be gentler also, and so not provide the degree of symptom relief menopausal women are looking for.

We've already referred to some of the herbs/vitamins recommended for easing the symptoms of menopause. Others include St John's wort and vitex agnus-castus, or chaste tree berries. St John's wort has been known to react with other medications, so check with your medical practitioner before taking it. In fact, this advice needs to cover any combination of pharmaceutical and herbal treatments.

There is also a large variety of plants which provide what is called *phytoestrogen*, a naturally-occurring oestrogen-imitating component. It's phytoestrogens that form the basis of bioidentical hormones, as we saw previously. In this group you'll find legumes such as soy, beans, flaxseed and chickpea as well as nuts and yams, wheat and oat bran and coffee, though this is by no means an inclusive list. Apples, pomegranates, cherries and carrots also contain phytoestrogen compounds.

The release of the results of the WHI trial in 2002, and the panic it caused about the use of HT prompted several studies into the efficacy of phytoestrogens in supplement form as an alternative to oestrogen replacement medications.

The results, however, were conflicting, with some studies showing phytoestrogen supplements helped, particularly with hot flushes, and others showing their use made no significant improvement for women whatsoever.

Again, like so many things to do with menopause, it's a case of 'give it a go yourself and see if it works for you. But do make sure, if you are working with more than one sort of therapy and therapist that you keep everyone in the information loop.

> One herbal cure many women swear by comes in the form of a herbal tea made with fresh lemon balm leaves. This tea is said to be great for reducing hot flushes, night sweats and palpitations. The official name of lemon balm is Melissa officinalis; it shouldn't be hard to find as it's easily grown.

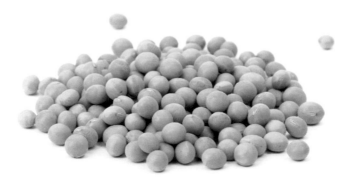

Q 69: My friend warned me against taking black cohosh. What's the latest information on using it?

Black cohosh is the root of a plant found in Northern America. It goes by the nickname 'black snakeroot' and is a phytoestrogen. For centuries, Native American healers used the herb for female reproductive problems, including menstrual cramps and bleeding irregularities.

In fact, black cohosh acts as an antispasmodic and an anti-inflammatory agent in muscles, nerves, and blood vessels, and is particularly effective for menstrual cramps and bleeding irregularities.

A 2008 study undertaken by the Flinders Medical Centre in Adelaide (Australia) recommended that care be taken with alternative and herbal medicines containing the herb. The study was prompted by the case of a 51-year-old Australian woman who developed liver failure while taking black cohosh. Her case was so severe she required a liver transplant.

The study examined another seven cases in Australia where liver problems could be linked with the use of black cohosh. In five of these, a liver transplant was required.

The study indicated that the herb appeared to be safe to use if taken for six months or less, but that further studies were needed and the community needed to be better informed about the herb.

According to Jean Hailes for Women's Health, more recent research into black cohosh has indicated it is safe to use, although some small concerns do still remain about its potential to cause liver damage.

In Australia the TGA has indicated, while it considers the herb suitable for use in complementary medicines, products containing it should still include a warning of the slim chance its use could cause liver damage.

Q 70: You mentioned a breathing technique as something new in the treatment field; can you give some more details?

Old and new, I think you could say.

What is known as *paced respiration* is one form of full, deep breathing that's been practised down the ages in disciplines such as yoga because of its benefits for health, calmness and general well-being. So, it's no surprise that deep rhythmic breathing is now being touted as a way to handle hot flushes.

A nine-week trial undertaken by Mayo Clinic (USA) researchers showed women who practised their breathing techniques for at least one, but preferably two 15-minute periods a day were able to reduce the number of hot flushes they experienced in a day by more than 50 per cent. Many women don't bother with two daily sessions, but simply start the breathing technique when they feel the beginning of a hot flush coming on, or when they have a quiet moment to themselves. The breathing appears to lessen both how long hot flushes last and their severity.

Paced respiration involves breathing deeply down into the diaphragm, which necessitates pushing out the stomach muscles. This inhalation should be slow and take approximately six seconds; the experience is like pushing out the stomach muscles. Then exhale slowly for six seconds, at the same time as pulling the stomach muscles in.

Detroit-based Professor Robert Freedman has studied women and hot flushes for more than 25 years and concluded that paced respiration could help reduce hot flushes significantly. He recommends in-and-out-breaths of five, rather than six seconds, but also advocates morning and evening sessions and the use of the breathing for the duration of a flush.

No one is quite sure how this concentrated type of breathing works to lessen the number of hot flushes some women experience, but it is possible it helps to cool the body by decreasing the amount of a hormone called norepinephrine in the body.

Q 71: Is there anything else worth considering?

A National Institute of Complementary Medicine (Australia 2010) report into complementary medicine concluded there was sufficient evidence to support the safety and efficacy of four complementary interventions. While these are not specifically for menopausal women, they are well worth considering for this time of life:

- Omega-3 fish oils for secondary prevention of heart disease
- Acupuncture for chronic low back pain
- St John's wort for mild to moderate depression
- A herbal combination used for osteoarthritis. This is sold as Phytodolor in the UK and Australia and is most likely found in the USA as Enzymatic Therapy.

Q 72: Do the experts have anything else to say about herbal remedies?

Again, we'll draw on the resources of Jean Hailes for Women's Health.

MYTH – Herbal remedies are safe because they're natural.
FACT – Up to 90 per cent of complementary medicines sold in Australia have potentially misleading labels.
ADVICE – Complementary therapy products, including herbal remedies, need to be treated the same as any other medication, and, just because something is 'natural' doesn't mean it's safe.

Complementary medicines need to be prescribed by a trained professional who can provide proper education about appropriate use, potential side effects and possible interactions with other medications.

So the advice is – make sure you tell your medical and/or other health and complementary medicine provider about all the medications you're taking – and that includes all complementary medications as well as pharmaceutical products.

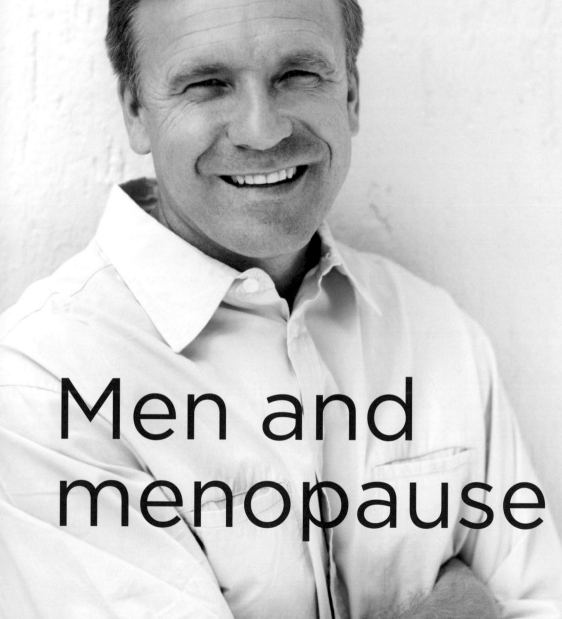

Men and menopause

Q 73: Do men have menopause?

Think 'menopause' and we think 'women of a certain age' but the biological clock ticks for men too – whether they like it or not. What is colloquially referred to as 'male menopause', however, is nothing like the dramatic change women go through. Rather, it involves a gradual decline in the production and levels in the body of male hormones, or androgens, and in particular of the hormone testosterone. This dropping of hormone levels starts long before most women start menopause.

Using the term 'menopause' for men is, therefore, a bit of a misnomer.

> The biological clock ticks for men too – whether they like it or not, but, for most men what is referred to as 'male menopause' is nothing like the dramatic change women go through.

The gradual drop in testosterone levels can be a genuine problem for perhaps one in three men in their fifties. It affects libido and sexual function and can lead to other health problems. For the rest of the male population, however, this slow decline in testosterone levels is just part of the normal ageing process, and a 'normal' man in good health might find by the time he's 80 his production of testosterone has dropped only by 30-35 per cent.

A man's 'hormonal health', however, starts to decline around the 30 years-of-age mark. That's when, for the majority of men, the production of testosterone starts decreasing. This rate of production decline varies enormously from man to man and family to family.

Testosterone is an important hormone for both men and women, but of course it has a much larger effect in men than it does in women. You could say it is in fact *the* male hormone. It's responsible in the growing male for the development of his testes and penis, for producing sperm and for his sex drive.

While a man can survive without testosterone, he won't have much of what we traditionally view as 'maleness' about him. And he's likely to have a whole lot of other problems as well, because testosterone plays a role in the development and on-going health of many bodily functions.

Testosterone has a role, for example, in strengthening bones, in stimulating the production of red blood cells in bone marrow, in the production of facial and body hair and the reduction of head hair; yes that old saying about men balding early being strongly sexed *may* have some truth in it. Testosterone levels also affect the growth and workings of the prostate gland, the 'voice breaking' that comes around puberty with the lengthening of the vocal cords and muscle strength. It stimulates the cells in the testes, assisting in the production of sperm, and it plays a role in a man's moods and even, at times, in his capacity to think clearly.

Decreasing testosterone levels is not always a bad thing ...

For the occasional man, it can come as a great relief to have lower testosterone levels in their system! One man in his early sixties – let's call him Bruce, claims the lessening of his sex drive in his fifties allowed him to experience real contentment for the first time in his life. His high sex needs in younger life had driven him to pursue women relentlessly – and while that was exciting, it had also been exhausting, and he had often felt as if he was not in charge of his life, but was being driven relentlessly by his own body. As his sex drive lessened, he found the time and peace of mind to start exploring different philosophies and ideas and has now fulfilled one of his life's dreams by writing two books.

Odd Spot

Obesity and low testosterone are a two-way bind for men, so it's worth starting the battle to fight the bulge the first time you have to let your belt out a notch.

Why? Because there's an intricate two-way relationship between declining testosterone levels and body fat. Too much body fat causes testosterone levels to drop, but low testosterone is also a cause of too much body fat. And it's not the sort of fat that's easily shifted; it's the deep subcutaneous abdominal fat that's associated with cardiovascular disease and metabolic syndrome, among other 'nasties'.

While there's lots of research going on around the world on testosterone replacement therapy, the best way to avoid the trap is to catch the problem at that first belt notch!

Q 74: What do men really need to know about menopause? Or should that read *what do women want at this time*?

The overt answer to the latter question is that women at this time of life want from their partners what they have always wanted from them: love, respect, care and time, to be treated equally, listened to with empathy (and not with an eye to problem-solving!), the odd compliment and an understanding that sometimes life can be a bit of a hormonal ride. I'm sure there's a great deal more, but that's as far as I plan to generalise on what's always private relationship stuff.

During menopause women want men to understand that the changes they're going through can be very disruptive for them and their own quality of life, not just their partner's.

Trying to sleep beside a woman who wakes in the night with hot flushes, hot and cold sweats and insomnia is no fun, but please try and keep it in perspective; it will pass, and in the meantime, it's 10 times worse for the one going through it. And if it's too bad, you can always go and sleep in the spare room or on the couch. Your partner can't escape the realities of her body's hormone roller-coaster quite so easily.

The unforeseen monsters

Sometimes women push their partners away for physical reasons; they don't want sex because they're too busy, too tired, too consumed coping with hot flushes, too busy coping with the emotional ups and downs that can come with fluctuating hormone levels.

But sometimes, women also push men away not because they can; they feel like they have an excuse. Menopause can be a time when much suppressed emotional stuff from the past comes bursting out like a volcano spewing lava. So past hurts and neglects, lost hopes and dreams, lack of care and attention, suppressed anger etc now come to the fore to be dealt with – or not, as the case may be.

What should men do? For goodness sake, take it seriously. Ignore it at your peril; it's not just a woman being emotional. If you want a future together with this partner, then find ways of working through these things together. Seek professional help, if needs be. Just don't ignore it – not if you want any life to be left in your relationship once this time of change is over.

Men really need to know that this is a phase, and it, too, will pass. But it will pass much more easily and almost inevitably with a better outcome if they try and understand what their partner's going through, do what they can to support her and take some of the burdens of everyday life off her shoulders.

I think there's been research that shows women find men particularly sexy when they're doing the vacuuming! I met a woman in my gym who is quite blatant about the fact she says to her husband that 'if you do the vacuuming, we'll have sex as soon as possible after you've finished'. She says (with a smile on her face) that it works every time!

Men also need to know what's happening in the woman's body and work with her to find ways that suit their changing sexual needs and circumstances. For example, they might need to start using vaginal lubrication so that dryness in the vagina doesn't cause the woman pain and prevent her from having pleasure.

Men need to be aware of their own changes too. Their sexual drive may have decreased – and that can give a couple the opportunity to put more quality and time into intercourse, to the benefit of both.

Q. 75: Can we say that falling testosterone levels are behind a man's so-called mid-life crisis?

The man suffering from a mid-life crisis has long been an easy target for humour; the butt of sports car, motorcycle, young chick and sex jokes.

But for the man who is experiencing the restlessness, pain and desire to break free from life's current restrictions that often hit in the early to mid-forties, life is no joke. It's a painful and often grief-filled time when desires, dreams and reality clash.

Is it caused by the slow decline in testosterone levels? It may play a part, but the mid-life crisis, or time of reassessment is more like a time when the realities of life all hit together.

For example, there's the knowledge that the rampant young sexual bull of former years has disappeared and no amount of wishing, wanting and experimenting is likely to bring him back. Also comes the realisation it may be too late to achieve the things in life he dreamed of when he was in his teens and early twenties. He may never make CEO, he may never climb the highest peaks in Africa or surf the curl at Jaws Beach in Hawaii. Or perhaps he has achieved many of his dreams, only to find his hard-won victories somehow seem empty.

Then, too, his responsibilities don't lessen; if he has children, they're probably reaching the expensive and challenging teenage years. Perhaps, too, his primary relationship has lost its satisfying edge – emotionally and physically – through busyness and habit. He sees his parents ageing and knows that's what lies ahead for him, without realising the peace and contentment that can come with those years.

He is, if he wants to let himself feel that way, trapped. He mourns his youth, but when he looks ahead sees nothing there to aspire to, no way forward that will bring him again the feeling of invincible life he had when he was young.

He's learning that he's mortal after all.

Difficult as this stage is for men, as well as their partners and others close to them, this is a natural cycle of life. Some men adjust and get on with living productive and fulfilling lives. Some men get stuck and choose to live in regret or bitterness for the rest of their days.

That said, the man going through this mid-life patch would be wise to have a full health check, just to make sure there's not some underlying cause for his malaise.

> The mid-life crisis can't necessarily be blamed on a man's hormones ... it's much more than that ... and painful as this time can be, it presents an opportunity for reflection and decision-making about what's really important in life, what dreams from youth still have validity, and what new dreams can be dreamt to drive the next productive stage of life.

Q 76: Is a man ever too old to be a father?

The answer is 'no, but ...'

At the same time as testosterone levels decrease, the potential increases for men to produce abnormal sperm and sperm with genetic abnormalities. The older the man, the greater the chance of their child being born with some sort of genetic abnormality. This is why now in most Western countries ultrasound technology is used to check the health of a child in utero, particularly those with older fathers – and in particular those with both mother and father aged 35 or older.

Having an older father – that's defined as one over 40 – has been linked to certain disorders in their children. These include dwarfism, autism spectrum disorders, schizophrenia and Down syndrome, with some studies finding fathers over 40 having an almost six-fold chance of producing a child with autism spectrum than men in their 20s and men in their 50s are three times as likely to father a child who develops schizophrenia.

But take heart – most men retain the capacity to produce healthy sperm throughout life, and therefore may be capable of fathering a child well into their later years. And, as Rmaajit Raghav says, healthy living and lots of practice do wonders for an older man's capacity.

Odd Spot

The world's oldest living father is said to be 96-year-old Indian man, Ramajit Raghav. Ramajit fathered a son in 2010 and a second son in 2012. He attributes his virility to his healthy lifestyle, which for him means eating mostly fruit and dairy products and having sex three or four times a night!

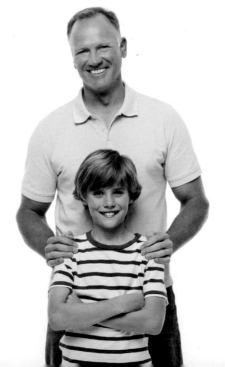

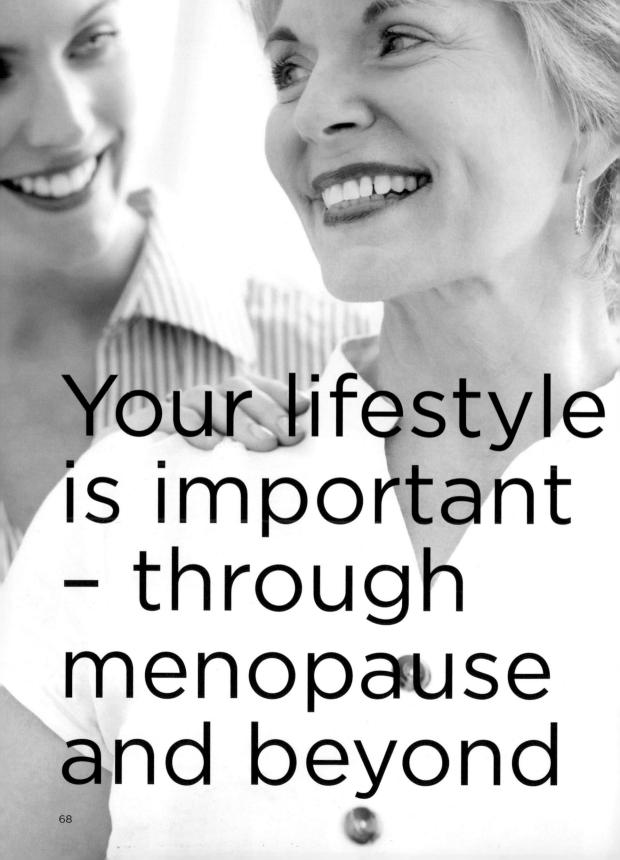

Your lifestyle is important – through menopause and beyond

What's new?

This is probably not new, but ...

- Women who exercise and follow a healthy diet cope better with menopause than those who don't.
- If you smoke, give it up if you possibly can. Women who smoke start perimenopause earlier, experience worse hot flushes and, apparently, don't respond as well to HRT in tablet form as their non-smoking sisters.
- Handling menopause requires a 'whole of life' focus.
- The mind/body link is important. How a woman thinks about herself generally and herself in relationship to menopause will affect her experience.

Q 77: You've called this section 'lifestyle' but what do you mean by that?

I'm going with my understanding - that it simply means 'the typical way a person chooses to live their life'.

Whether we like to accept it or not, the way we choose to live our lives affects our health, both in the short- and long- term. At the same time, our individual lifestyle is a product of what we've created in and with our lives as well as how we've responded to life circumstances. This applies whether we are rich or poor, in natural good health or not.

Lifestyle is also a product of what we believe is right or wrong for us, what we value and think is important now and in the future. All this, of course, is within the laws and constraints that living in our communities and countries imposes on us.

For example, our favoured lifestyle might include going to bed at dawn having played loud music all night. But we may not be able to live like this because of constraints imposed by people around us whose chosen lifestyles clash with ours, with theirs being acceptable to local authorities and ours being acceptable to almost no-one but ourselves!

So you could say, then, that 'lifestyle' covers a whole range of areas of life like health and body image, diet, relationships, work, creativity and interests.

The lifestyle picture is made more complex because our sense of self can be very caught up in our lifestyle choices, without us really recognising the connection.

Q 78: What do you mean by that?

It isn't the purpose of this book to go into how our minds work ... but, put simply, we each hold an image of ourselves in our subconscious and try, unconsciously, to match how we live to that image. That means, when we come to make changes to our lifestyle we're usually working to change the current image we hold of our 'reality', our 'self-image' in our subconscious. Changing self-image may take a lot of determination and will power!

What I'm really trying to say is that we can find it hard to change our lifestyles because of all these factors – and menopause is a time in life when lifestyle adjustments may well need to be made.

Q 79: But surely we have choice over most things in our lifestyles?

Indeed we do, but the older we get, the harder it can be to change aspects of our lifestyle that are not necessarily productive at our current stage of life.

The longer we've lived with habits e.g. the amount of exercise we take, or what we like to eat, the harder it is to change those habits that run counter to our best interests at menopause and beyond. Our preferences are programmed into our subconscious as our 'normal' and we have to re-program preference tapes about normality in our minds if we're to make lasting change.

There's one simple principle that governs lifestyle during perimenopause, menopause and the post-menopausal years in a woman's life – and that is that women who exercise and follow a healthy diet cope better with the changes that go on in their lives than those who don't. They also give themselves a better chance of protecting against other diseases such as heart disease and osteoporosis.

I said one simple principle, but I've just come up with a second one, or at least a corollary of the first – if you're a smoker, give it up if you can before you start perimenopause. Women who smoke start perimenopause earlier, experience worse hot flushes and, apparently, don't respond as well to HRT in tablet form as their non-smoking sisters.

Q 80: You previously mentioned heart disease and osteoporosis as post-menopause risks ... Are these things I really need worry about?

Earlier on we spelt out the best-known and some of the lesser-known symptoms of menopause. Some of these lessen or disappear altogether once menopause is complete. Others may linger for months or years. And some present challenges for the rest of a woman's life. Heart disease and osteoporosis fall into the last category, unfortunately.

Most post-menopausal women find their hormonal systems settle down a year or two after menopause and the mood swings that came with hormone changes settle down too. The decrease in oestrogen that a post-menopausal woman produces, however, can affect almost every part of her body. Vulnerability to acquiring heart disease and osteoporosis are two potential longer term outcomes of this reduction in hormone levels.

- Osteoporosis occurs because one of the roles oestrogen plays in the body is to signal to bone cells to stop breaking down. Reduce the supply of the hormone and the results are obvious. Women lose on average 25 per cent of their bone mass in the decade after menopause.
- The role oestrogen plays with coronary artery disease is thought to relate to its role in maintaining healthy cholesterol levels in the blood. Coronary artery disease happens when high levels of cholesterol lead to plaque building up in the arteries surrounding the heart, eventually blocking blood flow to the heart muscle. Many women find their cholesterol readings start to climb after menopause.

There are other longer-term effects of having less oestrogen in the system as we age as well; things like poor bladder function, loss of memory capacity and possibly an increased risk of Alzheimer's disease, loss of strength and muscle tone, and maybe degeneration of vision.

And then there's weight gain ... something most of us fail to avoid!

So, whether we like it or not, living a healthy menopause requires a disciplined lifestyle.

Heart palpitations may not be a message of doom
....
Heart palpitations are quite common at this time of life for many women. This may be tied up with the fact a hot flush can increase the heart rate by as many as 15 beats per minute while it lasts, or it may simply be the direct effect of fluctuating hormones, reducing oestrogen etc. The research isn't clear.

Whatever the cause, if heart palpitations are worrying you enough to see your medical practitioner be cautious that you don't accept a heart disease diagnosis without questioning it; palpitations may be a temporary symptom that rights itself after menopause. It wouldn't do to have to take unnecessary medications.

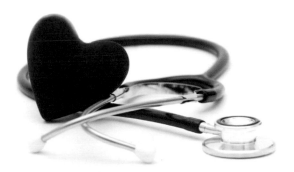

Q 81: This post-menopause picture is all doom and gloom as far as I can tell! Do I really want to go there?

Looks like I haven't sold you yet on the benefits of life after menopause, despite the annoyance of living with the symptoms of an ageing body ... That's a journey of discovery I hope you come to yourself, as I and many of my friends have.

But there's one simple piece of advice that will help prepare for menopause and improve your life afterwards. It's so important, I'll repeat it; get and keep yourself physically fit and eat a healthy diet. Physically fit means doing weight-bearing exercises, not just running, walking or other aerobic exercises.

Studies show that women who exercise and eat well by-and-large have an easier time physically, emotionally and mentally through the years before, during and after menopause.

Just swapping a diet high in carbohydrates, fat and highly processed foods for one with more protein, fresh fruit and vegetables and high quality fats is enough to improve a woman's well-being significantly.

Q 82: What about weight gain?

Forget the hot flushes and the night sweats, it's the slowly accumulating weight and the change in body shape that goes with it that worry many women most.

The unpalatable truth is that we women at menopause usually experience at least some weight gain, particularly around the abdomen. In fact, the majority of us find ourselves changing shape – with little we can do about it. Whereas previously we might have gained weight around the hips and thighs, now is settles around the mid-lower back and stomach. Those of us who once had waists can find ourselves now looking for them in vain!

Increased fat does have a purpose
....
Increased fat is one of the body's ways of coping with the drop in oestrogen supply from the ovaries. The body looks for alternative sources, and fat cells are one such source. So the body increases the conversion of calories/kilojoules into fat in order to access oestrogen. However, on the downside, overweight women usually have more severe flushes than those of normal weight!

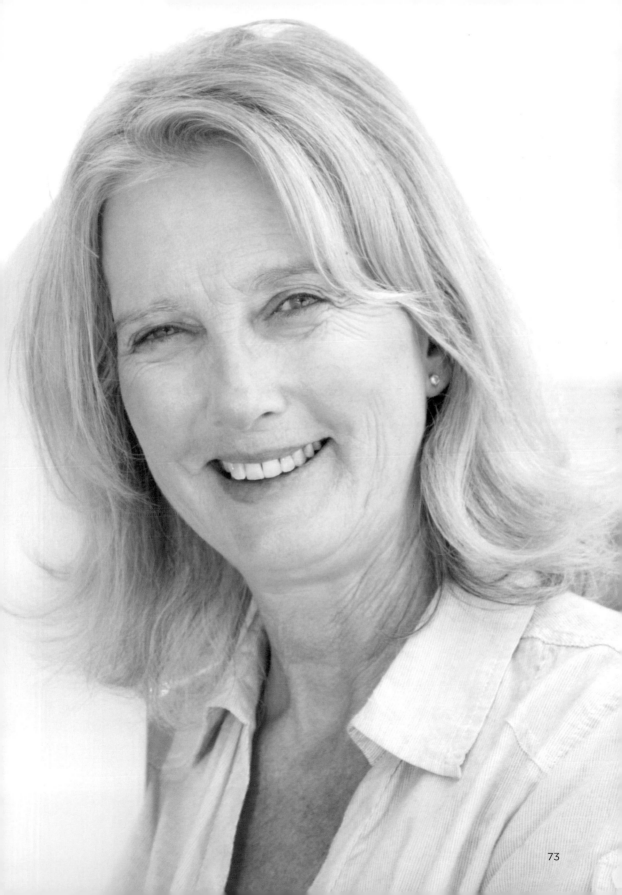

Q 83: Is oestrogen the culprit?

There are other hormones involved in weight gain as well as oestrogen. Lower levels of progesterone, for example, can lead to water retention in the body, while the decline in testosterone helps slow the metabolism. So, for many of us, what used to be a healthy amount of food on the plate now becomes overeating.

All this unfortunately is exacerbated by the fact that post-menopause many women also slow down their levels of physical activity. Some of us simply find it becomes harder to get ourselves motivated to exercise. For others their years of running around after a family are coming to an end, leading to less incidental activity in everyday life. We might be more relaxed now life is less stressful, and relax our eating controls as well. Other women can turn to eating for stress release.

The decline in testosterone is also responsible for decreasing women's muscle tone and muscle mass, which in itself contributes to weight gain. Testosterone helps the body to turn calories/kilojoules into lean muscle mass. Muscle cells burn more calories than fat cells do, meaning the more muscle, the higher our metabolic rate. Metabolism is the body's process of converting what we eat into what it can use and store – burning up calories/kilojoules as it does so. So the higher our metabolic rate, the fewer calories we have left to be turned into fat and deposited in places we don't want it.

Q 84: That's all very well, but what can I do about it?

I'll give some strategies shortly, but the first thing I want to say won't be popular, but here goes: *Hard as it may be to accept, some weight gain at menopause is a good thing.* Here we're talking about a few pounds/kilograms, not great heaps of weight. A rapid rise of two dress sizes, for example, should ring the alarm bells, whereas one dress size over a few years is not so bad, depending what size you started from, of course!

> The herb Chinese angelica, or dong quai, is said to help with balancing postmenopausal hormones. It also works, apparently, in reducing hot flushes. You can use it as a tea, in a tincture or as a capsule, taking 3-4g per day.

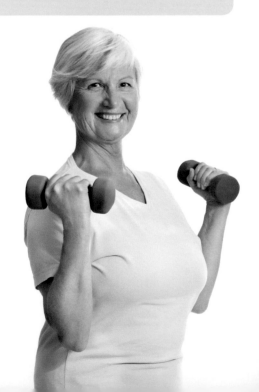

Q 85: Why would some weight gain be good?

There are several reasons, not all of them justifications! Some extra weight:

- Is natural. It's happened to women lucky enough to have sufficient food in mid-life down the ages.
- May be part of some women's genetic programming! Check out your mother and grandmothers etc for an idea of your genetic inheritance.
- Helps you fend off or reduce your chances of getting osteoporosis and various other illnesses. If you do become ill, having some reserves of muscle and fat helps the healing process no end; it gives you energy reserves to draw on.
- For some unexplained reason can help lessen the severity of hot flushes and menopause-related anxiety. This may have something to do with more of that great balancing hormone oestrogen being accessible from the fat cells, but here I'm only guessing.
- Overweight women usually have more severe flushes than those of normal weight!

But too much weight gain is no lightweight issue.

Q 86: What problems can excess weight gain cause?

Excess weight gain can signal various problems for a woman's life satisfaction and health.

She might, for example, have developed insulin resistance, a process whereby the cells of the body can't fully utilise the energy available for repair and functioning. That energy then becomes stored as fat. More protein and green vegetables in the diet help, in tandem with muscle-building or resistance exercise.

Or it might be a sign of too much stress in her life. The body can't distinguish between one sort of stress and another, and will go into 'famine prevention mode', turning every available calorie/kilojoule into fat for storage to cope with tough times ahead.

Then again, excess weight might signal a whole lot of other health problems, including diabetes – so best advice is head to your health practitioner for a check-up.

The keys to maintaining a healthy weight

- The first and most obvious one is to try not to put too much extra weight on in the first place. It's much, much easier to prevent weight gain happening at menopause than it is to take those unwanted pounds/kilograms off afterwards!
- Eat a balanced diet including sufficient protein, unrefined carbohydrates, fruits and vegetables. Avoid refined sugars and trans-fats.
- Don't go on crash diets and don't lose too much weight. Crash diets will encourage your body to switch on its survival mechanisms and slow down your metabolism. When you stop the diet (as we all inevitably do), you'll have set yourself up for more and more rapid weight gain. And should you actually succeed in becoming thin, and keeping the weight off, then you will be increasing your chances of developing osteoporosis. I can vouch for the 'no crash diets' message, having lost many kilograms, mostly from around my middle, and then seen them return, even though I only changed one small thing in my diet. Ho hum.
- Become more active – and that means including a variety of activities. Aerobic exercise such as swimming or jogging or very fast walking will boost your metabolic rate, and weight bearing activities such as resistance work in the gym, walking and cycling increase muscle mass and improve fat burning, as well as helping prevent osteoporosis.
- If you find yourself feeling bloated, best to cut down on alcohol and drinks containing caffeine, especially coffee, as these exacerbate fluid retention.

Q 87: I've heard or read all of this before. Isn't there anything new you can add?

Not only have you probably heard, or read, it all before, if you're like me you've probably also come across a whole lot of misinformation you'd have been better off not hearing or reading at all.

I do, however, think there are a couple of new things in this lifestyle area. The first one is the push for women to focus on overall healthy living rather than on different aspects of health such as

getting fit, for example, or losing weight, or preventing osteoporosis. So it's a *whole of life focus*, rather than just dealing with things one at a time and in isolation.

The other thing that's new, or emerging anyway, is something I mentioned earlier – and that the link between the mind and the body and the effect this has on a woman's experience of menopause and growing older.

Perhaps another way to put that would be that this emerging area for research explores the possible link between how we think about menopause and how we think of ourselves (our self-image) and the literal experiences we actually go through in the transition.

Q 88: Can you please explain what you mean?

I guess it's counter-intuitive, but if we're looking at making lasting change for the better, we need to start with how we think, not how we eat or exercise. This is how we can develop the will-power we need if we're to make, and persist with, productive change.

So, I'll ask you, do you see yourself as a woman who is active every day? *Think fitness, moving, activity – not weight loss.*

We need to *do activity every day* in order to make on-going change that helps alter our self-image. As we stick with our activity schedules, slowly our subconscious picture of ourselves changes; it aligns itself with a picture of yourself as a woman who is active every day, eats well etc. That, in turn, helps us become a person who is active every day and eats a good diet. And so it goes. Every time you stick with your activity schedule and go out walking, working out etc, it becomes easier to maintain your commitment to exercise and living a healthy lifestyle.

This mental focus is vital. Our subconscious hates dissonance; that is, it does not like your inner picture of yourself, your self-image, to be at odds with the outer reality. In the example I'm using, the reality is that you are now a person who exercises and eats well, while the image your subconscious clings to is of you before you began this regime. So, if you keep up your schedule, good diet etc then your self-image will change.

The picture you have of yourself in your subconscious will come to reinforce how you now live your life as an active person ... and so you should find it becomes easier as time goes by to keep on living in this active, healthy way. What you're doing with this self-image stuff is strengthening your will, that is, your ability to carry through on what you set yourself to achieve.

Why go to the bother in the first place? Because starting and maintaining activity for at least 30 minutes a day, every day (well, maybe you can allow yourself one day off per week!) will keep the weight down and improve your sense of well-being.

It might take a bit of re-organising your daily schedule and some co-operation from others such as your partner and perhaps children. It may mean finding a supportive person to exercise with. It may mean developing the habit of getting out of bed an hour early, summer and winter.

But, whatever you need to do to make it happen, it will be worth it.

Q 89: Will taking HT make me put on weight?

Simple answer: contrary to popular belief, the research shows we can't blame HT. We have to look elsewhere for those extra pounds/kilograms.

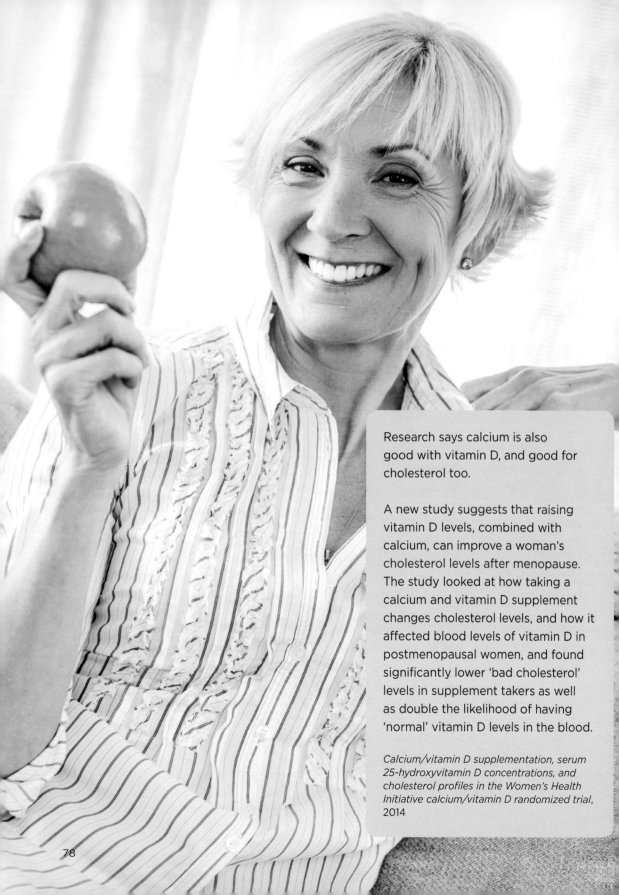

Research says calcium is also good with vitamin D, and good for cholesterol too.

A new study suggests that raising vitamin D levels, combined with calcium, can improve a woman's cholesterol levels after menopause. The study looked at how taking a calcium and vitamin D supplement changes cholesterol levels, and how it affected blood levels of vitamin D in postmenopausal women, and found significantly lower 'bad cholesterol' levels in supplement takers as well as double the likelihood of having 'normal' vitamin D levels in the blood.

Calcium/vitamin D supplementation, serum 25-hydroxyvitamin D concentrations, and cholesterol profiles in the Women's Health Initiative calcium/vitamin D randomized trial, 2014

Q 90: You keep mentioning a good diet, what might that be for a woman during menopause?

Not only do I think diet is important both pre and post menopause, I also think it's so important I'm including a list of what you might call menopause 'superfoods' (see box). There's also a selection of recipes at the back of this book to help you include these healthy foods in your diet.

The basics of a good diet during and after menopause, however, are much the same as for any other stage of life, unless you have special needs. A good diet includes adequate lean protein such as salmon, high-fibre carbohydrates, lots of fruit and even more vegetables, low-fat, low-sugar and salt, healthy oils (e.g. olive rather than palm oil), and low-fat dairy products.

Add to this foods rich in calcium to counteract bone mineral loss, and consider taking a calcium supplement, or combined supplement including calcium and magnesium.

Also try adding foods that are a good source of phytoestrogens, as these will help with preventing or ameliorating hot flushes. As we listed before, this food group includes soy products such as tofu and soy milk, plus some cereals/dried seeds – flax seeds and oil, chickpeas, lentil, barley and cracked wheat, for example.

Limit your intake of the sorts of foods that are high in calories/kilojoules, but are poor sources of nutrition. Top of the list has to be soft drinks, followed closely by cakes, biscuits, chips and crisps.

Many women suffer from inadequate levels of Vitamin D as they go through menopause and beyond. In fact, research has shown that older women living in care are the group most likely to suffer from its lack. Vitamin D is vital for healthy bones as it helps the body absorb calcium, and the best source of it comes via exposure of the skin to sunlight for at least a few minutes every day. It can be found in some foods including oily fish, eggs and liver. Milk and other dairy products in some Western countries are also supplemented with it.

Check whether your diet has sufficient Vitamin E as well. This has been found to help in some cases of severe hot flushes. Vitamin E is found in green leafy vegetables, wheat germ and various oils (safflower, soybean, and corn oil, for example).

Make sure you add some of these foods and food groups to your diet wherever you can - they're said to be the menopause 'superfoods':

Flaxseeds and flaxseed oil
Extra virgin olive oil
Beans
Lean meat
coldwater fish (including salmon)
Broccoli
Yams
Soy, fermented soy, tofu
Whole grains and nuts
Yoghurt (low fat and sugar)
Berries

It protects red blood cells and enables the body to use Vitamins A and C more effectively.

Perimenopause is a time to check the levels of iron in your blood as well, particularly if you are experiencing increased blood loss. Many women become anaemic around this time, that is, they have insufficient iron in the blood to produce the amount of haemoglobin they need.

Meat, particularly red meat, is a good source of iron, but so too are eggs, nuts and legumes, so check your diet for an adequate amount of these foods.

Q 91: Lack of sleep is making me ill. Is there anything I can do apart from taking sleeping tablets?

Thousands of women would sympathise with you. The fatigue, tension and irritability that come with sleep deprivation during menopause often get mistaken for symptoms of menopausal hormone change itself when, in actual fact, they are simply the result of lack of sleep.

If you were a young mother with a new baby suffering the same effects of lack of sleep no-one would question your right to be cranky and you'd attract much more sympathy. But such is the unfairness of life!

The fact men suffer much less from insomnia or sleep difficulties than women do at most stages of life simply adds to this unfairness.

Sleep patterns change during menopause for two reasons:
- Firstly, hot flushes and night sweats are very disruptive to peaceful sleep, even when they don't wake a woman up. They make us restless and uncomfortable, and
- Secondly, at least one study has shown that night-time hot flushes and sweats tend to come when we are in deep REM sleep. REM sleep is the sleep we can't do without if we're to feel refreshed in the morning.

Sleep cycles change as we age; we seem to need less and it is more disrupted. It's not yet known if this is to do with changing hormone levels, though this is probable. Some women find it increasingly hard to fall asleep, but the more common pattern is to fall asleep easily but find yourself awake perhaps three or four hours later, and then have trouble getting back to sleep. Waking might be caused by our bladders being less flexible than they used to be, but that's not necessarily the main reason.

I have a couple of strategies that work for me. Firstly I realise I need perhaps an hour's less sleep than I used to, so I tend to go to bed an hour later, and often sleep through. And I make the nights I do wake the time I allocate myself to do all my lighter reading until the next sleep cycle kicks in.

As for surviving it, I'm afraid you may have to work out your own strategies for this. Many of my friends take sleeping tablets, others practise relaxation techniques both before bed and when they wake in the night. Some women claim acupuncture works as well.

Cutting down on caffeine and alcohol in the evening hours is also important, as these definitely disrupt the quality of sleep. Personally I know that if I even have half a glass of wine within four hours of bedtime I'll go to sleep okay, but I'll be awake again instantly three hours later almost to the minute – and have great trouble getting back to sleep. So, it's just not worth it, unfortunately.

I have one married friend who finds she can do a couple of hours' uninterrupted writing in the wee small hours and cherishes her awake time.

So, changing sleep patterns need not be all bad! Beyond medicating to change them, there's not a great deal we can do about them anyway.

Q 92: My mother tells me she suffered from severe headaches when she went through menopause. Is that common?

It's quite common for women to get headaches around the time of their normal periods, due to the change in hormone levels, and certainly some women do claim to suffer headaches and migraines during menopause.

Experts link headache onset to fluctuations in oestrogen levels, rather than consistently low oestrogen, and so they may lessen or stop altogether once menopause has been completed.

Treatment options are as varied as the type and cause of the headache or migraine, so usually needs the intervention of your medical practitioner. In some cases the answer is an oestrogen supplement taken at a certain phase in the menstrual cycle.

Q 93: Is there anything else unpleasant I should know about?

We're getting to the end of the list, but there are a couple more worth mentioning. One is that body odour seems to change. I find this one hard to explain but I have noticed it myself, even though the change is subtle. So, it's something you will need to be aware of for yourself; you might be quite different and come through menopause smelling of roses!

It would seem there's nothing much we can do about this change beyond being ultra-aware of everything to do with personal hygiene.

Some women also notice their skin and hair get dry. While this seems to be a natural part of ageing, particularly for those of us who live in countries with hot summers, it also has something to do with reduced levels of oestrogen.

The advice is obvious; protect your skin, use moisturisers and hair conditioners, balancing it all with the need to have some sun exposure each day so our Vitamin D needs are met.

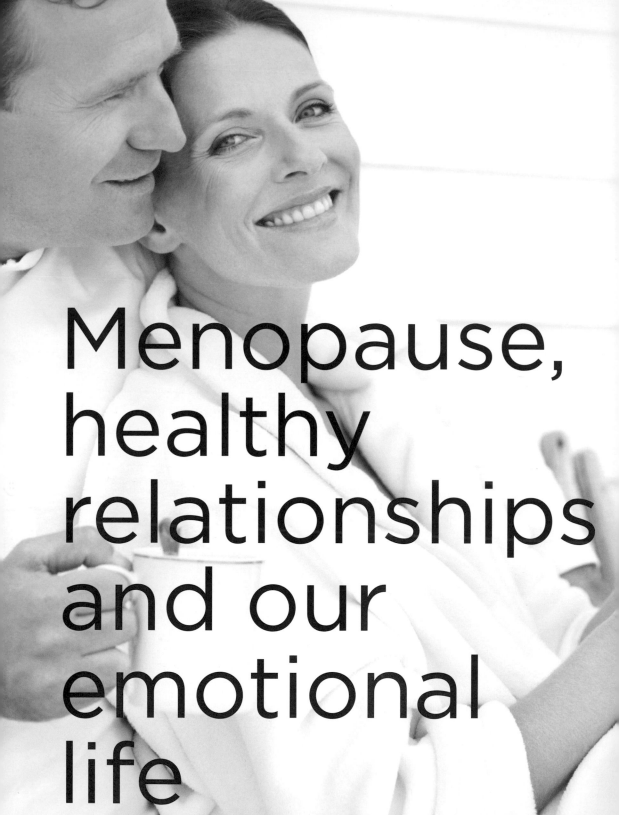

Menopause, healthy relationships and our emotional life

What's new?

- Expanding the conversation about menopause and relationships to include life-stage/whole-of-life questions and spirituality, not just hormones and physical health. That means expanding the conversation to bring in partners and their issues, needs and expectations as well.
- Recognising the connection between physical and psycho-social factors and how these can influence a woman's experience of menopause.
- Accepting that making the best of the menopause transition and life afterwards may well require women to be courageous!

Relationship crises are a common side effect of menopause – and blaming women's hormonal changes is an easy tactic. But, like all things to do with the complexity of human nature and change, it's not that simple.

Like every aspect of the menopausal journey, the emotional ride during the whole menopause process and beyond is unique to each woman. Some of us sail through happily and are relieved to get to the other side, others find their mood swings upset every relationship, in particular those with close partners; yet others find themselves under a cloud of depression, anxiety and grief that fails to lift even when menopause is over.

Menopause is not just a simple story of dealing *physically* with hot flushes and night sweats etc. Our menopausal experience is also a story of our emotional/psychological journey as well.

According to Australia's Jean Hailes for Women's Health, medical and other health practitioners are starting to understand the link between psycho-social factors and a woman's physical experiences of menopause.

In other words, what's going on in our everyday lives – psychologically, socially and culturally – also can have an influence on how we experience the menopausal time of change in our lives, and, of course, the opposite is true as well. What we experience also affects our experiences day to day.

Q 94: Okay, I can accept that in principle, but what sort of things are you talking about?

When I talk about psycho-social factors I'm referring to things like:

- Whether we've previously been sufferers of mood swing problems or depression, or whether they just are unwelcome visitors at this time.
- Where we're 'at' in life – for example, do we have children leaving home (the 'empty nest' syndrome), are we coping with teenagers (the 'oh I wish at times I did have an empty nest!' syndrome), whether I'm partnered or not …
- Our roles in life – worker (happy, stimulated, frustrated, bored), balancer of work, home and parenting, mother of daughters, sons, 'sandwich carer' (caught looking after both older and younger generations), student, volunteer, etc.
- How we think about menopause and ageing. This can be influenced by our family's attitudes, by the norms of our culture e.g. whether older women are respected in our society or treated as past their use-by date, our ideas of sexuality and whether our sense of self is tied up with being seen as 'a sexy or sexual woman' etc. So different social and cultural expectations affect how we think about menopause and ageing.
- Our body image – this is a fraught area for many of us, especially in Western cultures where the worship of 'the young, the perfect and the fit' is insidious and causing all manner of psychological problems for young girls and indeed women of every age. But bodies do age – and there's little in the finality we can do about it.
- Our sexuality and libido – again a complex area and we'll go into this in much more detail shortly.
- Our support systems, including our family and friends; nothing like having people you can talk to whom you can trust not to judge you or to gossip about you. With luck, many of us will have such support people within our family and friendship groups.
- And last, but by no means least, our relationship with our partner. Is it robust and supportive, distant, lost its intimacy … what's going on in our partners' lives at this time, and so on.

Q 95: Now it's my turn, as writer, to ask you the reader a question or two; are you a positive or negative person? Do you look forwards in life or do you look backwards?

Why do I ask? Because how we look at things affects what we experience during and after the menopause life transition.

Whether we're a glass half full or glass half empty person, our attitude will influence how we cope with life's challenges during this time. Our emotional wellbeing and how much we yield to the mood swings brought on by hormone change depend *at least to some extent* on our attitudes.

What we think, we create. Our emotional responses follow on from our thoughts. Difficult to accept and work with, but true nonetheless. It's the same principle at work as when we need to change our self-image to reinforce lifestyle change.

A 2009 Australian study[8] supports the half-full/half-empty theory. It revealed that women with high emotional intelligence seemed to approach menopause more positively and experience less severe stress and psychological distress than women in the research group assessed to have a lesser degree of emotional intelligence. These women also appeared to suffer less severe menopause symptoms and have better physical health.

The researchers concluded that that "women who expect menopause to be a negative experience or are highly stressed or distressed may be more likely to experience a more negative menopause".

Emotional intelligence is defined as the ability to identify, use, understand and manage emotions in positive ways that enable us to relieve stress and defuse conflicts.

It also enables us to empathise with others, overcome challenges and communicate and interact with others effectively.

Q 96: Does other research support these findings?

A 2011 study undertaken in Turkey[9] also investigated the attitudes of a group of women and their male partners to menopause.

A second aim of this study was to investigate whether a relationship existed between these attitudes and the women's experience of symptoms including depression and anxiety.

The study concluded that, at least among this group of women and their partners, the majority were positive about menopause and their experience of it. The study also identified a possible link between the severity of menopausal symptoms and partners who were not so positive.

But of course, it's a chicken and egg situation; it's impossible to identify which comes first – a woman having severe symptoms and a partner responding negatively to that, or a negative partner influencing a woman's attitude and, possibly, therefore the severity of her symptoms.

An earlier US study[10] seems to indicate attitudes in the Western world may differ from those found in the Turkish study. The US research concluded women were more positive about menopause than their male partners. The women also thought they experienced more symptoms than their partners perceived them as having. Both men and women, however, found that having a positive attitude was related to reporting fewer menopausal difficulties.

The other significant finding in this study was that post-menopausal women were more positive about menopause than either those experiencing perimenopause or those who had gone through surgical menopause.

So, I'm not alone in thinking there's life after menopause!

Q 97: I guess that a lot of the other psycho-social factors you mentioned also swing around attitude?

I guess so, but I don't think we can be too prescriptive here. If you come from a long line of women who have had a difficult time at menopause that doesn't mean you can sail through yours just by having a positive attitude! Genetics and a whole range of other physical and health-related issues will play their part in your experience too.

But being happy with yourself and the roles you fill in life and believing that you have value and what you do matters and makes a difference to others does give you a foundation of well-being that often promotes health and leads to experiencing less intense menopause symptoms.

Body image is a difficult part of menopause for many Western women, influenced by media images and marketing emphasis of youth and the perfect body shape etc. The

messages are pervasive in our cultures, even when we're older and 'should' have more sense.

I put 'should' in quotation marks because it usually refers to some external rule or regulation that's we've adopted … that doesn't really belong to us, but which we allow to govern our thinking in some way.

Menopause can affect a couple's relationship because for many women body image does matter. Some women start to feel ugly and undesirable, and that of course, has an effect on the couple's sexual relationship and intimacy.

But bodies change – and some of the most beautiful women I've ever come across are obviously in their post-menopausal years. Their beauty comes from the fact they are happy in themselves and content with their lives and their inner beauty inside shines through the outside wrinkles.

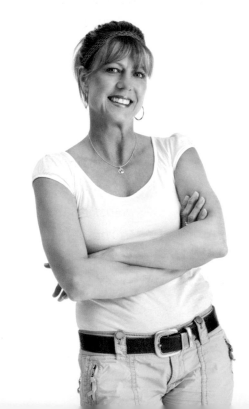

The body-image thing and vanishing middle-aged woman

"How we think about our changing bodies – our body image – can be one of the hardest psycho-social aspects of menopause to deal with. It's not just that the body changes; this change often forces us to confront how much we have come to rely – consciously or unconsciously – on ourselves being seen and treated as desirable, sexual people of obvious fertility.

"I remember one day when I realised I had reached that point in life: it was a real shock. I'm not saying that as a younger woman I was a head-turner – by no means. But as a woman I could always sense when interest, in my case from the opposite sex, came my way whether I was looking for it or not. Whatever the feminists might say, for me that is just part of the interplay between the genders; it need not mean anything more than that.

"This particular day I was walking down the street in a major city, and I realised that I had 'become invisible'. It sounds stupid, but I had the sense that no longer did anyone notice I was there. I'm not talking only about men not noticing, I'm talking about anyone noticing. When women are younger, other women notice them too: it's not just men who do. But I, in my late-forties, had become an invisible middle-aged woman.

"It took me a while to get over that, but now I relish the freedom. I no longer care what people think, what or if they notice when I'm within their orbit ... I can be me without any of that other stuff tying me down."
Peggy M. Bath, UK

Q 98: Are you really saying that when it comes to coming through menopause positively we really need to have good relationships?

That summarises it pretty well – relationships with trusted others and, even more importantly, with ourselves. Any relationship difficulties a woman experiences can affect her moods at a time when she's also dealing with menopause. What a time for many women to be parenting teenagers!

It is no secret that relationship crises are a common side effect of menopause, and we're not just talking about a woman's primary relationship with her partner. All relationships are affected and many need re-negotiating.

Why? Because menopause isn't just about stopping menstruation; it's the start of a whole new phase of life. And the most important relationship that needs to survive menopause and come out stronger on the other side is a positive and loving relationship with ourselves.

Remember what's being unleashed
....

Menopause can unleash a woman's confidence and creative juices! Now that she doesn't have the reproductive hormones taking up or obscuring her drive for creativity and achievement, a post-menopausal woman can be a power to be reckoned with – and just at a time when her partner may want life to start slowing down. Many a woman's life turns 360 degrees, as new careers are pursued and vocations followed. It takes strong relationships with committed partners to re-negotiate the potentially stormy years of the later forties and early fifties as women's long-sublimated desires are released. This energy can be like a volcano demanding release.

Many women refuse any longer to accept injustice and partnerships that aren't equal. This means around one-third of partnerships in the Western world don't or can't manage to renegotiate their relationships. Many women are no longer willing to put their own needs aside in order to support and nurture. Some couples stay together, papering over problems as and how they can; others head to the divorce court. And of those divorces, seven out of every 10, so the statistics say, are initiated by women.

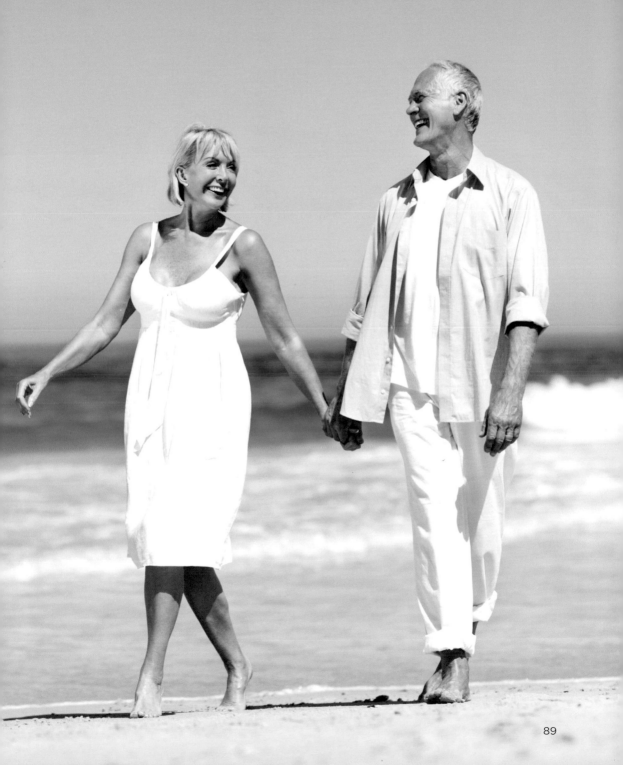

The primary relationship for most women is their intimate partner. Leaving aside the question of sex for the moment, it seems that once again how we and our partners think is vital. Menopause can put the soundest relationship under considerable strain, both during the lead-up phase and afterwards.

There are several reasons:

- The physical changes and discomforts that may be part of the process. What we can say here is a menopausal woman's partner often needs patience and understanding and the willingness to set aside, or be willing to negotiate about, their own needs.
- While the decline in male hormones is a slow process, menopause represents an obvious and intense, much more sudden, change for women. *Both partners need to see their partner with new eyes at this time of life.*
- For some relationships the things that have served as glue holding a couple together have naturally run their course. Menopause may serve as the final stressor in such relationships. For example, children are older and independent and the couple have little left in common together.

All relationships, whether they're strong or not, will need re-negotiating during the menopausal transition.

Q 99: If you had to advise a couple about their relationship during menopause, what would you say?

I think that I'd say something about the need to keep on working on your relationship in the same way you need to have been working on it since Day One – caring for each other, being sensitive to each other's needs, sharing experiences, making time to listen talk and be intimate, understanding the need for time alone away from each other, valuing each other and supporting the other person's interests and sense of purpose in life.

There are some physical things that need to be, and can be, accommodated as long as people have patience and respect for each other. So, here at last we come to *sex and menopause.*

A 2010 UK (University of Sheffield) study found most menopausal women's attitudes to sex at this time of life had more to do with social and psychological factors than with declining hormones, although it is hormones which usually get the blame for declining action in the bedroom.

A couple's quality of relationship, other life interrupters (e.g. caring responsibilities) and the interest of the woman's partner in sex, sex drive and capacity to achieve and maintain an erection were all viewed as important contributors to women's interest in and satisfaction with their sex lives during and after the menopausal years.

So we can intuit that boredom, lack of time and tiredness, anxiety, poor sexual and other relationship incompatibilities all affect sexual satisfaction at menopause as at any stage of a relationship.

Nonetheless, hormone changes can – but don't have to – affect a woman's libido. There is some research that shows for some women the desire for sex actually increases at this time, despite the decline in hormone levels.

The reasons for differences are as varied as the women.

I had a beloved aunt who told me when she was in her sixties that sex just got better and better! And an elderly friend, now well in her nineties, told me when her husband died about 20 years ago that the thing she missed most was sex.

We, male and female, may need to work a little harder to achieve orgasm, but hey, what the heck ...

So, I guess, what this research is saying is that, if you have a good relationship before the menopause years, there's no reason that will not continue through these years and beyond – provided you're willing to keep working on it. And you may even find your new freedom includes the freedom to explore and reinvigorate your sex lives. The changes a good partnership goes through can lead to lots more genuine care and intimacy – as distinct from sex – and that turns many of us women on!

Then again, is anyone questioning the assumption that it's important for women to want and need to remain sexually active in later middle age and beyond? For some it might be a great hindrance to finding satisfaction in life, while for others it may not matter so much, and for others, giving sex a looooong rest may even come as a relief! A whole range of responses is perfectly fine as far as I'm concerned. The energy used in sexual activity does not get lost if it's not expended for that purpose, it just gets used differently.

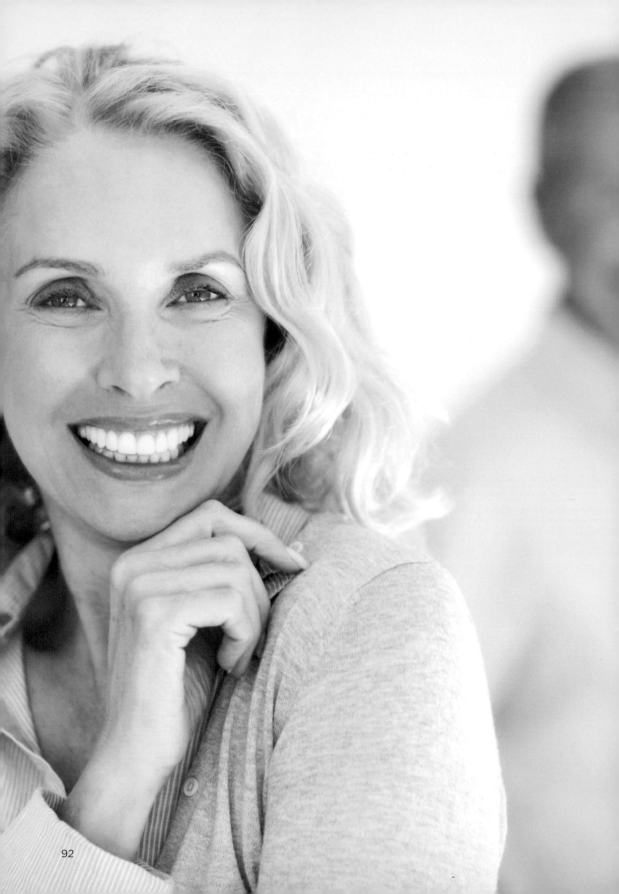

Q 100: What are the main challenges when it comes to sex?

Menopause does bring many challenges in the area of sexual activity, including:

- Lack of interest in sex is a genuine physical problem for many women (though some are happy for it to be so!). This goes in tandem with a difficulty in becoming sexually aroused and can have a hormonal basis. Libido drops substantially across the menopause transition usually because of the drop in oestradiol. This change has a name – female androgen insufficiency syndrome – which is a way of defining how androgen deficiency in women would be manifested. Treatment in the form of hormone replacement is available.
- Various physical conditions, such as vaginal dryness, which is a fact of life for most women at menopause and beyond, unless they're on some form of HT. Vaginal dryness and thinning of the vaginal walls can make sex painful, but this can be eased by the use of various oestrogen-based creams and other lubrications. The good news too is that lots of practice keeps the blood flowing where it's needed most! Painful sexual intercourse goes by the name dyspareunia and is something that really needs to be discussed with your medical practitioner.
- Other physical conditions might also interfere with interest in sex; chronic pain, anaemia, underactive thyroid gland and various infections, such as thrush or urinary tract infection fall into this category. Again, the advice is to seek medical or other professional assistance.
- And then there's the fact that by the time many women hit their menopausal years, their partners may have begun having their own problems with getting and maintaining an erection – and this requires tolerance and much else from both partners if they're to adjust and have an on-going, loving sexual relationship. Some relationships just don't have that in them anymore; others flourish on the intimacy.
- I also have to include physical appearance too. We've already mentioned that many women worry about their own attractiveness and how their partners feel about them, whether they still find them attractive etc. Nobody talks much, however, about whether women still find their partners attractive. The research shows men are, unfortunately, more likely to 'let themselves go' than women as they hit middle age, which can be a 'turn-off' for partners. I don't have any advice to give here ...

> Post-menopausal women may be at risk of sexually transmitted diseases, especially if they are exploring new relationships and choose not to use condoms. But then again, don't we assume menopause frees us from thinking about such annoying things as condoms? Unfortunately not, and the statistics now say the rate of STD infection and diagnosis is growing rapidly among people aged over 60, and especially over 70.

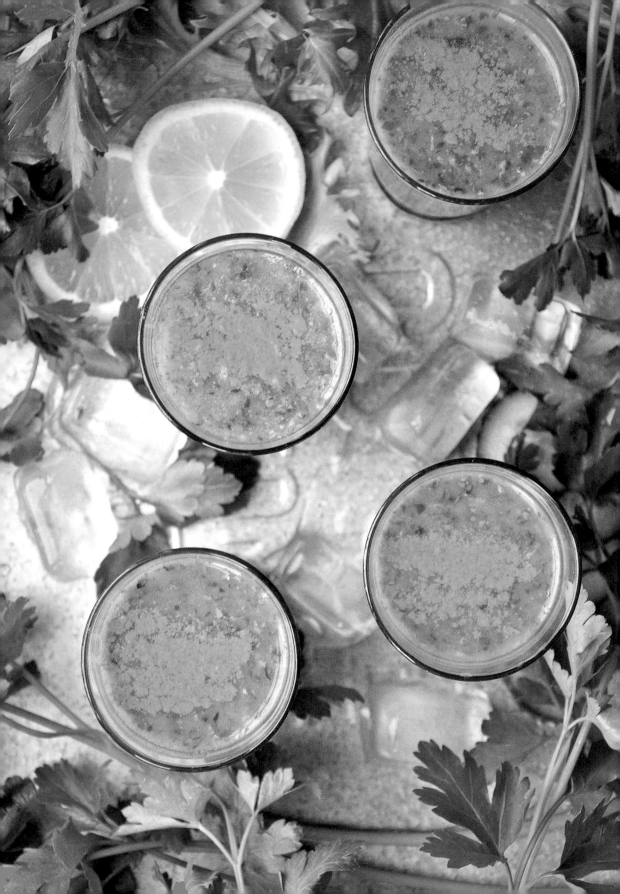

Wake me up smoothie.

Serves 2

1 cup (65g) baby spinach (or kale, silver beet)
1 ripe banana (frozen for extra creaminess)
½ an avocado
1 small cucumber
½ inch piece of fresh ginger root
Handful of fresh parsley
1½ cups (375ml) water
¼ cup (60ml) lemon juice (fresh)
Handful of ice
Ground turmeric for dusting

1. Chop all ingredients up into similar sized chunks.

2. Combine spinach, banana, avocado, cucumber, ginger, parsley, water, lemon juice and ice in a blender and blend on high until smooth and creamy.

3. If more liquid is needed add in additional water a little at a time until desired consistency is reached.

4. Pour into two glasses and top each with a dusting of ground turmeric. Alternatively, add the ground turmeric or a 1 inch piece of fresh turmeric at step #2.

Naked bean burgers with sweet potato crisps

Serves 4

1 can (400g/14oz) kidney beans
1 can (425g/14oz) black beans
3 spring onions (scallions)
1 tsp sea salt
1 tsp black pepper
2 tsp smoked paprika

1 medium beetroot
1 avocado
1 medium sweet potato
Kale or lettuce leaves to serve

1. Preheat the oven to 180°C/350°F.

2. In the bowl of a food processor combine the kidney beans and black beans.

3. Slice onions and stir through the mixture with sea salt, black pepper and smoked paprika.

4. Divide the mixture into 4 and roll each portion into a hamburger patty shape. Place each patty on a baking paper lined tray. Bake in the oven for 20 minutes, set aside to cool before removing from the tray.

5. Grate the beetroot using a box cutter or food processor.

6. Slice avocado and drizzle lemon juice over the top to stop the avocado browning.

7. To make the sweet potato crisps, use a vegetable peeler to peel thin slices or chip off little crisp-size bites.

8. Lay the sweet potato on an oven tray lined with baking paper. Drizzle extra virgin olive oil over the top and sprinkle with a pinch of sea salt. Bake in the oven for 10 – 15 minutes or until crisp.

9. Assemble the burger by placing the patty on a small pile of baby kale or lettuce leaves, top with avocado and the raw shredded beetroot. Sprinkle the sweet potato chips over the top.

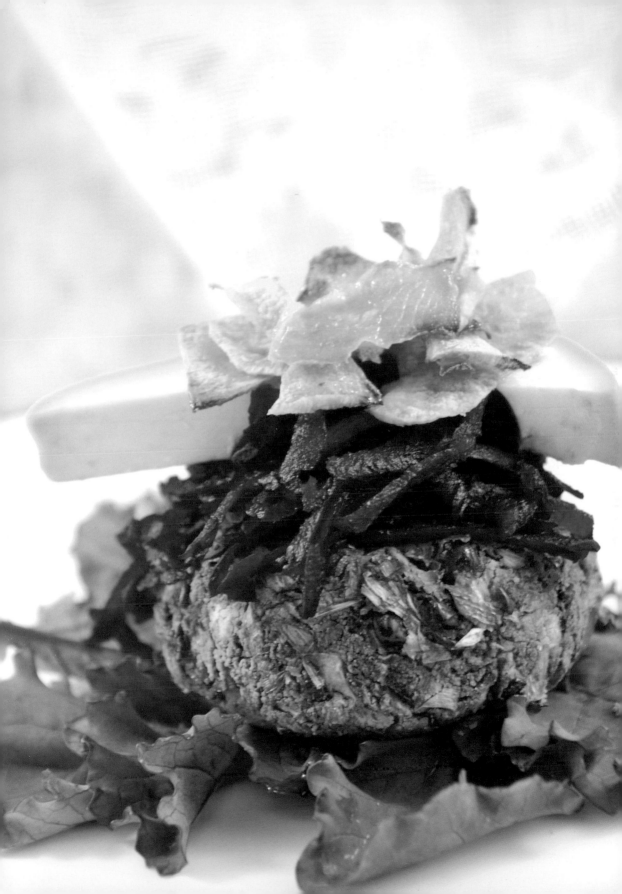

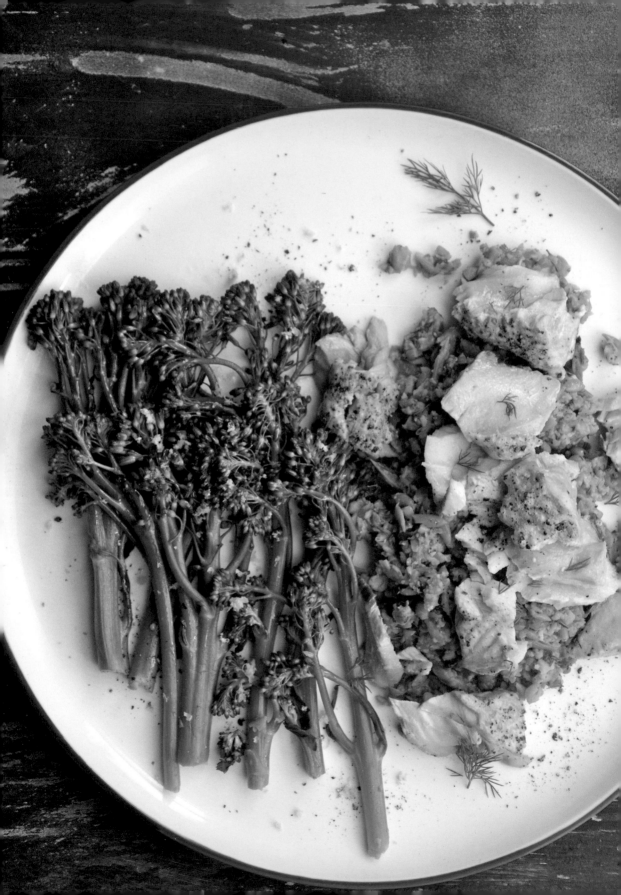

Pan seared salmon with dill pea mash

Serves 2

2 medium salmon fillets
1 tsp sea salt
1 tsp black pepper
Zest of 1 lemon
1 tsp paprika
Extra virgin olive oil
3 cups (385g) peas
250g/9oz broccolini
1 tbsp unsalted butter
¼ cup (25g) fresh dill, finely chopped

1. Season each salmon fillet with sea salt, black pepper and lemon zest. Drizzle with extra virgin olive oil and set aside.
2. Heat a frying pan over a medium heat and add the salmon skin side down. Cook for 4 minutes each side.
3. While the salmon is cooking, steam the peas and broccolini until tender then stir through the butter and dill. Set the broccolini aside and mash the peas roughly with a fork or using a food processor to create a creamier mash.
4. Serve the salmon fillets on top of the pea mash and alongside the broccolini. Squeeze fresh lemon juice over the top.

Spiced Broccoli, Kale & Lentil Bowls

Serves 2

½ tsp ground cumin
½ tsp chilli flakes (or fresh chilli)
¼ tsp cinnamon
¼ tsp ground coriander
¼ tsp ground fenugreek (optional)
Sea salt
1 garlic clove, crushed
1 inch piece of fresh ginger root, grated
1 head of broccoli (including stem), cut into small chunks
1½ cups (100g) kale, roughly chopped
1 can (400g/14oz) cooked lentils
2 tbsp coconut oil
2 tbsp natural yoghurt or coconut milk
Zest of ½ lemon
¼ cup (30g) walnut pieces (optional)

1. Combine all spices in a bowl.

2. Lightly steam broccoli and kale and set aside.

3. Drain the lentils and rinse thoroughly under water.

4. In a pan over medium heat add the oil and spice mix, cooking gently to release the aromas.

5. Add the broccoli, kale and lentils and coat with the spices. Heat through.

6. Serve the spiced broccoli, kale and lentils with natural yoghurt, lemon zest and walnuts on top.

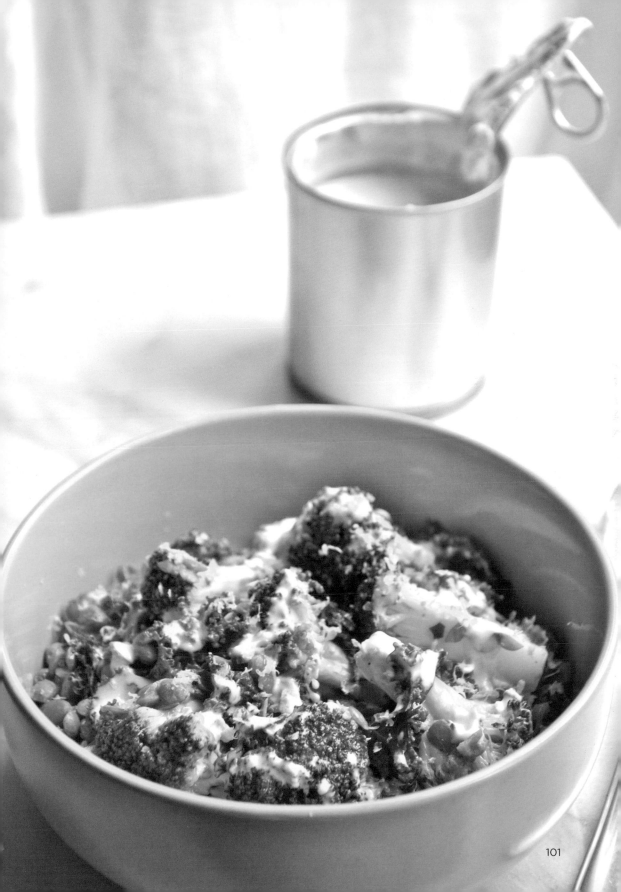

Spicy beef and spinach curry

Serves 2 – 4

500g/1lb sirloin or rump steak
½ Spanish (red) onion, finely chopped
1 inch piece of fresh ginger root, finely grated
4 garlic cloves, crushed
3 red chillies (any variety), finely chopped
1 green chilli (any variety), finely chopped
1 cup (250g) diced tomatoes
2 cups (500ml) beef stock (plus more stock or water as needed)
300g/10oz baby spinach leaves

1. Slice beef into thin strips and sprinkle lightly with sea salt.

2. Heat up a large cast iron pot or saucepan over a medium heat. Add a drizzle of extra virgin olive oil and add onion, ginger, garlic and chilli. Sweat for 3-5 minutes. Add the beef, tomatoes and stock, stir and reduce the heat to low.

3. Simmer for 45-60 minutes until the beef is tender, checking every 15 minutes and adding additional stock or water as needed. Add spinach leaves 5 minutes before serving.

4. Serve on a bed of cooked rice or mashed sweet potato, with a side of steamed green vegetables and natural yoghurt to dissipate the heat if needed.

Conclusion

When I was growing up, I can never recall menopause being called by that word, its true medical descriptor. Instead, it usually went by the euphemism 'change of life', as if this were the only real change ever taking place in a woman's life.

As for men's slow transition, this wasn't acknowledged openly at all. Perhaps people simply took the ageing process as a given, and didn't try to slow it down as so many of us attempt to do these days.

When I think about it, it seems like I lived my childhood and teens in the dark ages! The introduction of the contraceptive pill happened in the early-mid 1960s and led to a revolution in how both women and men could live and control their lives. Over the subsequent years this seems to have enabled a much more open and freer attitude to all things relating to bodies, sex and reproduction.

I suspect the rapidly developing field of assisted reproduction may herald changes of similar magnitude as time goes by; what they might be, I can't imagine, but the technology is already freeing some women from the restriction of time-based fertility through egg and embryo freezing and storage.

Regardless of what we may achieve through science, let's not forget that behind these physical bodies we give so much time to tending, behind our desires and goals, our feelings and our day to day continuum of thoughts, we have a very different clock ticking. It's one we have little control over.

I'm referring of course to our natural life clock, the pattern of our inner life development. I would call it our spiritual clock, but that's not a word everyone is happy with.

It's the clock that says there's a natural stage at life for many things. We may be physically capable, for example, of defying menopause and having a baby at 50 or 60, but this places us profoundly out of step with the inner development patterns of life. Our years beyond 50 and particularly beyond 63-64 ask us to expand our vision from the constancy of the everyday and to find outlets for our subtle urge to serve and be of use in new ways.

There's a rhythm and pattern to life and menopause is a natural part of it. So let's live through it as best we can, getting the right help if we need it, and enjoying life at whatever age and stage we find ourselves.

Index

References

1. Flint M, *The menopause: reward or punishment?, 1975*

2. Jean Hailes for Women's Health, *The Rumours aren't True*

3. Jean Hailes for Women's Health, *The Rumours aren't True*

4. From research undertaken by Jean Hailes Foundation for Women's Health

5. Jean Hailes for Women's Health, *The Rumours Aren't True*

6. Jean Hailes for Women's Health

7. Cummings, Herald, Moncur, Currie, Lee: *Women's attitudes to hormone replacement therapy, alternative therapy and sexual health: a web-based survey*, Dr Gray's Hospital, Elgin, UK

8. Griffith University, *Stress, psychological distress, psychosocial factors, menopause symptoms and physical health in women*, Bauld & Brown

9. *The attitudes of menopausal women and their spouses towards menopause*, Aydin School for Health Sciences, Adnan Menderes University Aydin, Turkey

10. *Attitude toward menopause among married middle-aged adults*, Department of Psychology, Western Illinois, University 2002